KT-469-023

SECTION 4 | HIV AND THE PRACTICE TEAM — 85

SECTION 5 | QUICK REFERENCE — 95

SECTION 6 | SUBJECT INDEX — 117

INDEX OF PHOTOGRAPHS

Forewords

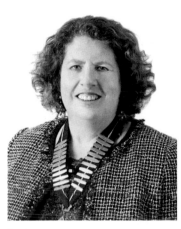

**Professor
Maureen Baker**

Antiretroviral therapy has transformed the management of HIV into that of a chronic condition. Early diagnosis has long term health benefits and allows cost-effective management, not to mention the avoidance of distressing and serious medical conditions. However, late diagnosis of HIV is associated with increased morbidity and mortality and although the proportion of patients diagnosed late has been falling, progress is slow: from 56% in 2005 to 40% in 2014.

Antiretroviral therapy also radically reduces transmission of the virus: if the patient is on the correct regimen, and taking it correctly, their risk of transmitting it can fall to close to zero. However, annual new diagnoses in the UK remain stubbornly at around 6000. The benefits of early HIV diagnosis are clear, but too many people living with HIV remain undiagnosed.

This booklet will give you and your team a number of ideas about how to increase HIV testing and improve diagnosis in both symptomatic and asymptomatic patients in your practice. The guidance takes a pragmatic, 'GP-centred' approach and never loses sight of the fact that HIV – like so many important conditions we need to be able to detect – is comparatively rare. Many HIV associated conditions ('indicator conditions') are common in their own right – shingles or seborrhoeic dermatitis, for example – and the challenges presented are not glossed over.

This short booklet offers helpful advice and ideas for the primary healthcare of patients with HIV in the general practice setting. It gives key points about antiretroviral medication including the signposting of invaluable, reliable, external sources of information to strengthen safety and quality when prescribing additional medications.

It's a resource by GPs – and for GPs. I can strongly recommend it.

Professor Maureen Baker
Chair of Council
Royal College of General Practitioners

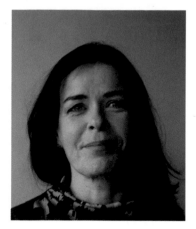

Silvia Petretti

I was diagnosed with HIV over 19 years ago at the age of 30 and I would have never expected to be alive today, at 50 and to grow older with HIV. A good relationship with my GP and primary care close to my home is incredibly important for my health. My GP surgery has always been a welcoming and friendly place in my local community where I can get treatment and support for everyday ailments from eczema to back pain. Up to now they have been very efficient in providing me also with yearly PAP tests and flu jabs, but I know that as I grow older my GP will play a bigger role in keeping me healthy.

With a growing population of people living with HIV who live longer and age with HIV, the role of primary care in managing our health and promoting our well-being is ever expanding. As I have worked supporting others with HIV at Positively UK over the past 16 years, I am aware that people with HIV can often be nervous about accessing care from their GPs, and that the GP may not always have all the information they need to support us.

Moreover GPs can play a crucial role in enabling people to test for HIV early. Sadly I have sometimes seen people being diagnosed very late, in spite of having been to see their GP several times with opportunistic infections which are tell-tale signs of HIV. This has often happened to older women, maybe because the doctors didn't perceive them to be at risk of HIV, or perhaps because they didn't feel comfortable and confident talking about sexual behaviour and HIV with an older woman.

Therefore I welcome this booklet as it can increase confidence and skills around HIV testing, treatment and care among healthcare providers in our communities. I also see this booklet as a useful tool that we as patients can promote and share with our doctors to improve our care.

Silvia Petretti
Deputy CEO
Positively UK

Preface

About this booklet

The number of people with HIV infection continues to rise. While there is still no cure and no vaccine, current treatments are life-saving and prevent onward transmission of the virus. A fifth of those with HIV infection in the UK have yet to be diagnosed, even though many will be using primary care and other medical services.

This booklet provides essential information for GPs, practice nurses and other members of the primary healthcare team on:

- HIV and the consequences of infection
- the clinical diagnosis of HIV in primary care
- HIV testing and prevention strategies in primary care
- the management of those with HIV – with a primary care focus

About MEDFASH

MEDFASH (Medical Foundation for HIV & Sexual Health) is an independent charity dedicated to quality in HIV and sexual healthcare. Originally established by the British Medical Association, MEDFASH has been supporting health professionals and policy-makers with educational resources and guidance since 1987.

Other MEDFASH publications include *HIV TIPs (HIV testing in practice)*, an educational web tool for general practice, *HIV for non-HIV specialists: diagnosing the undiagnosed*, a booklet for healthcare professionals working in secondary care, and *Standards for the management of sexually transmitted infections (STIs)*, produced with the British Association for Sexual Health and HIV (BASHH). MEDFASH has also managed the delivery of the Sexual Health in Practice (SHIP) training programme for GPs and practice nurses in a number of London boroughs.

About the authors

Dr Philippa Matthews MBBS FRCGP was a GP in central Birmingham and London for many years, and still keeps her hand in with regular locum work in Kings Cross, London. She is currently working in rural KwaZulu-Natal, South Africa, where the HIV prevalence is amongst the highest in the world. She is Clinical Lead for sexual health for Islington Council, and also Clinical Lead for HIV and Sexual and Reproductive Health for the RCGP. She has produced a range of written, online and face-to-face materials teaching about HIV and sexual health, with a strong focus on sexual history-taking and communication skills.

Dr Sara Madge MBBS MRCGP works as an associate specialist at the Royal Free Centre for HIV Medicine in London, having worked in HIV/AIDS since 1992. She has a background in general practice.

Dr Surinder Singh BM MSc FRCGP is a senior lecturer at UCL and a GP with a long-standing interest in HIV and AIDS. He has been a senior partner in a thriving practice in Deptford, London, since 1992. He was a member of the original Independent Advisory Group on Sexual Health and HIV, established in 2002 as part of the Government's national strategy for sexual health and HIV in England. Latterly he has been a performance assessor for the GMC.

Dr Nick Theobald MA MSc MBBS trained in general practice in Bath and Wiltshire and was a GP principal in Swindon for nine years. He was associate specialist in HIV/genitourinary medicine at Chelsea and Westminster Hospital and Imperial College, London, with responsibility for undergraduate and postgraduate education until 2014. He now works freelance in medical education and coaching.

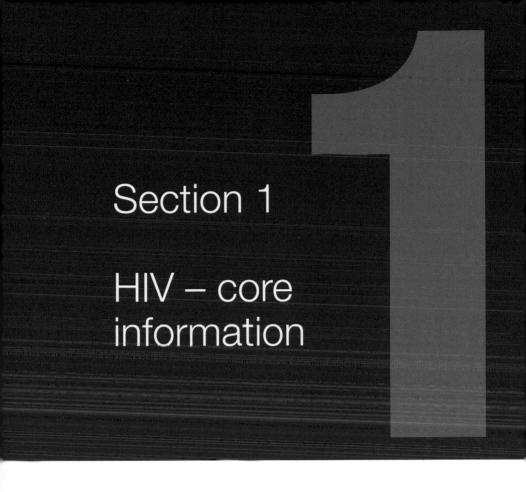

Section 1

HIV – core information

IN THIS SECTION

HIV – core information

For those who need an update on HIV, its effects and how it is treated and prevented.

HIV in the UK: the figures

1. How common is HIV in the UK?

Human immunodeficiency virus (HIV) continues to be one of the most important communicable diseases in the UK, with over 100,000 now infected and over 6,000 new diagnoses a year.

2014 figures show that men who have sex with men (MSM) were the group most affected by HIV in the UK with an estimated 45,000 (one in 20 MSM aged 15–44) living with HIV, and over 3,000 new infections a year in this group (see figure 2). The second largest affected group were Black African men and women, with around 30,000 (one in 56 men and

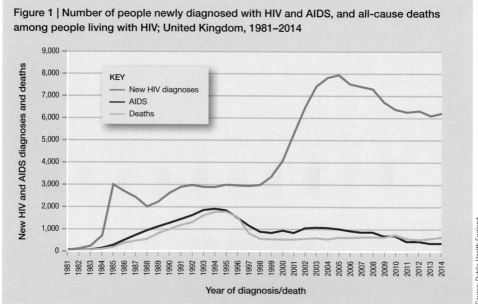

Figure 1 | Number of people newly diagnosed with HIV and AIDS, and all-cause deaths among people living with HIV; United Kingdom, 1981–2014

Source: Public Health England

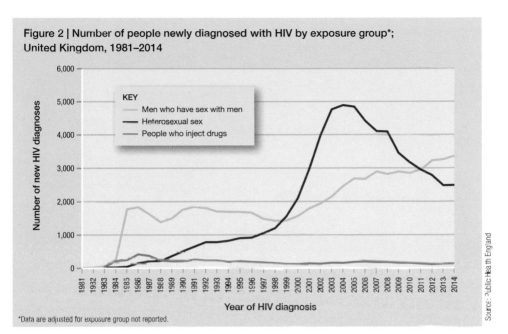

Figure 2 | Number of people newly diagnosed with HIV by exposure group*;
United Kingdom, 1981–2014

*Data are adjusted for exposure group not reported.

Source: Public Health England

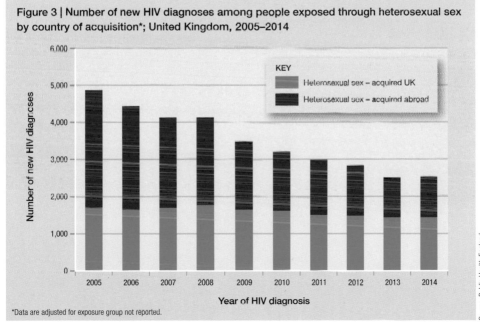

Figure 3 | Number of new HIV diagnoses among people exposed through heterosexual sex
by country of acquisition*; United Kingdom, 2005–2014

*Data are adjusted for exposure group not reported.

Source: Public Health England

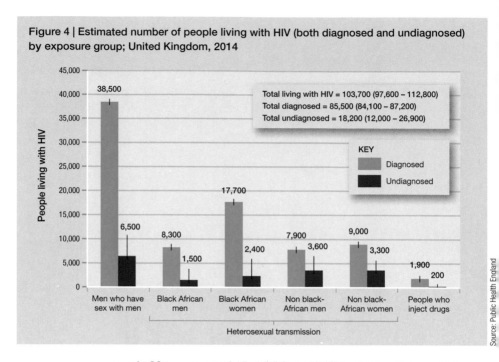

Figure 4 | Estimated number of people living with HIV (both diagnosed and undiagnosed) by exposure group; United Kingdom, 2014

Total living with HIV = 103,700 (97,600 – 112,800)
Total diagnosed = 85,500 (84,100 – 87,200)
Total undiagnosed = 18,200 (12,000 – 26,900)

KEY
Diagnosed
Undiagnosed

Source: Public Health England

one in 22 women aged 15–44) living with HIV, reflecting the very high prevalence in the region of origin of this population.

Whilst Sub-Saharan African countries are recognised to have a very high prevalence of HIV, many other countries from which UK residents originate or to which they travel have a substantially higher prevalence than the UK. These include the countries of the Caribbean, parts of Eastern Europe and the Far East, and parts of South America. For more information see *Global AIDS Update 2016* on the global epidemic from UNAIDS. However, of <u>new</u> diagnoses made in the UK in heterosexuals in 2014, three in five were thought to have been acquired here (see figure 3).

2. The impact of treatment on death rates in the UK

There has been effective treatment for HIV since the mid-1990s. Antiretroviral therapy (ART) and other interventions have resulted in a dramatic reduction in the number of deaths among those diagnosed with the infection (see figure 1). If diagnosed in a timely fashion, HIV is a chronic condition with an increased risk of long-term morbidity but normal or near-normal life expectancy – mirroring other important long-term conditions, such as diabetes.

3. Undiagnosed HIV

Undiagnosed HIV matters for two important reasons. Patients will benefit more from early treatment with ART; many of those undiagnosed have advanced infection (see Late diagnosis, below). In addition, the risks of onward transmission of infection are much higher in those not treated, particularly those who are not aware they have HIV. Based on anonymous seroprevalence surveys, it is estimated that almost one in five people living with HIV (17 per cent, 18,100) remains undiagnosed (see figure 4) and it is a public health priority to reduce this fraction.

4. Late diagnosis

HIV-related morbidity and mortality are concentrated among the two-fifths of people living with HIV who are diagnosed late. Although individuals diagnosed late can do well, late diagnosis is associated with a tenfold increased risk of death within one year. There is evidence that a significant proportion of people diagnosed late have been seen in general practice within the year prior to their diagnosis. Some presented with, in retrospect, HIV-associated symptoms but were not offered an HIV test (see page 105 for a list of indicator conditions).

Early diagnosis improves health outcomes and is cost-effective, as timely initiation of ART leads to fewer episodes of acute serious illness, including both AIDS and non-AIDS related events. The use of antiretrovirals (often referred to as ARVs) also lowers infectivity to a highly significant degree and greatly reduces the risk of transmission to others.

Monitoring HIV in the UK: how is it done?

1. Measuring diagnosed HIV infection

Public Health England (PHE) and Health Protection Scotland (HPS) collect information on newly diagnosed HIV infections, AIDS diagnoses and deaths based on voluntary case reporting by laboratories and clinicians. In addition, annual surveys of adults attending for HIV-related care provide a geographical distribution of diagnosed cases as well as information on uptake of ART. This information is available on the PHE and HPS websites.

2. Measuring undiagnosed HIV infection

The Unlinked Anonymous Seroprevalence Surveys provide data on the prevalence of HIV infection in selected adult populations (pregnant women, sexual health clinic attendees and injecting drug users). Blood samples taken in participating centres for other reasons are irreversibly unlinked from patient identifying information and tested anonymously for HIV. The surveys help monitor trends in the prevalence of both diagnosed and undiagnosed HIV infection in these settings. Participants are always offered a personal HIV test as part of these surveys.

The virus and the natural history of HIV infection

1. The human immunodeficiency virus

HIV is a retrovirus, which preferentially infects immune system cells – particularly a class of T lymphocytes called CD4 cells (also known as T helper cells). It is present in an infected person's blood and in other body fluids, including semen, vaginal secretions and breast milk.

For more on primary HIV infection see page 28

A flu-like illness is common in the first few weeks after infection and may be mild or quite severe, although some patients remain asymptomatic. During this phase called 'primary HIV infection' (also known as HIV seroconversion illness) there are large amounts of replicating virus and the patient is very infectious.

Once the symptoms of primary HIV infection subside, an asymptomatic stage of infection begins. There is a wide variation in the time it takes to progress to symptomatic disease and the individual may be well for many years even though the virus is actively replicating. Ultimately the normal levels of CD4 cells can no longer be maintained and as their numbers decline the immune response is undermined. At the same time, the amount of virus in the blood ('viral load') starts to climb.

2. The consequences of HIV infection
Opportunistic infections

For more on clinical problems caused by HIV infection see page 31

If untreated, infection with HIV results in the development of HIV-associated opportunistic infections (OIs). Fungi, viruses, bacteria and other organisms that are usually controlled by a healthy immune system can all cause OIs. Some, such as candidiasis or herpes zoster, are more common in the immunocompromised. Others, such as *Pneumocystis* pneumonia (PCP), cause infection in the immunocompromised only.

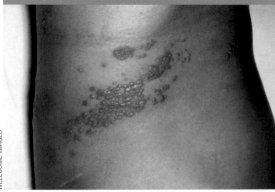

Herpes zoster. Commoner in those who are immunocompromised, this condition is one of the opportunistic infections associated with HIV.

WELLCOME IMAGES

Malignancies

Some malignancies are associated with untreated HIV infection including Kaposi's sarcoma (KS), non-Hodgkin's lymphoma and carcinoma of the cervix. When diagnosed in an HIV-positive patient, these cancers classify the individual as having developed AIDS. Other cancers including cancer of the lung, Hodgkin's lymphoma, anal cancer and some skin cancers may also occur at a higher rate in the HIV-infected patient. Several of these malignancies are themselves associated with viral infections, for example KS and human herpesvirus 8.

Metabolic abnormalities and cardiovascular risk

People living with HIV are at higher risk of metabolic abnormalities including dyslipidaemia and insulin resistance. HIV is associated with inflammation and immune activation. The precise mechanisms and role of therapy versus other risk factors in this are still debated. HIV-positive individuals are also at a higher risk of several age-related morbidities including chronic kidney disease and low bone mineral density.

Direct effects

HIV itself causes a flu-like illness in the weeks after infection. In advanced disease it may cause wasting, diarrhoea and neurological problems, although these may also be caused by OIs.

3. Acquired Immune Deficiency Syndrome (AIDS)

The term AIDS was coined before HIV was identified in order to help classify and monitor a new medical condition. There are now much better measures of disease progression (see pages 17–19) and it is more common to refer to 'advanced HIV disease'. Thus 'AIDS' now has limited value with respect to prognosis. It is, however, still used as a category in epidemiological surveillance and also in resource-poor countries.

A patient with HIV is said to have AIDS when they develop certain conditions. As well as the malignancies described above, infections leading to an AIDS diagnosis include: *Pneumocystis* pneumonia (PCP), cytomegalovirus (CMV), progressive multifocal leucoencephalopathy (PML), *Mycobacterium avium intracellulare* (MAI), cryptococcosis, cryptosporidiosis and toxoplasma encephalitis.

Tests and clinical markers of HIV infection

1. Combined HIV antibody and P24 antigen tests

The most commonly used test to diagnose HIV looks for both the HIV-1 and HIV-2 antibodies as well as a protein of the virus, the HIV p24 antigen. These 'fourth generation' tests are an improvement on previous HIV tests which looked for antibodies only, because of the reduced window period (see below). The combined test should be available to the great majority of GPs in the UK and this can be confirmed with the local lab. In the event of a positive result a second sample is requested for confirmation. These tests gives no indication of disease progression.

2. The window period

Antibodies to HIV typically appear four to six weeks after infection, but this may very occasionally take as long as eight weeks. The p24 antigen can be detected in a blood sample for a short period after infection, normally appearing within 10 days to five weeks, but it rapidly becomes undetectable once antibodies to HIV start to develop. The period between becoming infected and antibodies developing is commonly referred to as the window period. Tests which rely solely on HIV antibody measurement (such as some point of care tests and self-testing kits) may therefore miss early infection. See box for current guidance on the window period for HIV tests (adapted from British Association for Sexual Health and HIV (BASHH) guidance)

USEFUL INFO
(Adapted from BASHH/Expert Advisory Group on AIDS (EAGA) Statement on HIV window period, 14 November 2014)

- Accredited diagnostic laboratories in the UK use 'fourth generation' tests for HIV. These test for HIV antibodies and p24 antigen simultaneously in venous samples, and will detect the great majority of individuals who have been infected with HIV at 4 weeks after exposure.
- Patients attending for HIV testing who identify a specific risk occurring less than 4 weeks previously should not be made to wait before HIV testing as doing so may miss an opportunity to diagnose HIV (in particular acute HIV infection during which a person is highly infectious). They should be offered a laboratory 'fourth generation' HIV test on a venous sample and be advised to repeat it when 4 weeks have elapsed from the time of the last exposure.
- A negative result on a fourth generation test performed at 4 weeks post-exposure is highly likely to exclude HIV infection. A further test at 8 weeks need only be considered following an event assessed as carrying a high risk of infection.
- Patients at ongoing risk of HIV infection should be advised to retest at regular intervals.
- Patients should be advised to have tests for other sexually transmitted infections in line with advice on window periods for those infections (see BASHH guidelines). Patients at risk, who are not immune to hepatitis B, should be immunised.

---

3. Polymerase chain reaction (PCR) tests

These quantitative assays are a form of Nucleic Acid Amplification Test (NAAT). They are not often used as an initial diagnostic test for HIV in adults as they are expensive and can risk a high false positivity rate in the absence of laboratory interpretation. However, they are the preferred test of specialists if primary HIV infection is suspected and the antibody/antigen test is negative.

4. Rapid HIV tests

Rapid HIV tests (also called point-of-care tests (POCTs)) generally test for HIV antibodies only, although some now also test for antigen. Antibody-only tests have a window period of 12 weeks before becoming positive. Oral fluid or pinprick blood samples are used, and a test result can be given within minutes of the specimen being taken. The specificity of rapid testing devices is lower than that of laboratory tests and, notably in low prevalence settings, this may result in some positive results being false positives. It is essential that all "reactive" POCT results are confirmed with a conventional blood test.

POCTs give fast results when a sick patient presents to the Emergency Department or a woman of unknown HIV status is in labour. They are also used in community outreach testing, in free home sampling kits, and in DIY self-testing kits, the sale of which was made legal in the UK in 2014.

POCTs are used for HIV screening in primary care in some areas. GPs wishing to use POCTs should discuss this with their local genitourinary medicine (GUM) or HIV specialist and virology lab lead.

5. CD4 lymphocyte cell count (CD4 count or T-cell count)

The CD4 count is an indicator of the degree of immunosuppression in those infected with HIV. In healthy, non-HIV-infected individuals the CD4 count is usually above 500 cells/μl, although some have naturally lower CD4 counts. CD4 counts are variable – for example, if someone has a cold or has recently had an immunisation. Therefore overall trends are more important than single readings.

The CD4 count declines at an average rate of 40–80 cells/μl per year in those with untreated HIV, but some infected individuals progress faster than others. There is wide variation in the time it takes to progress from primary infection to symptomatic disease (see figure 5). Patients with a CD4 count of below 200 cells/μl are at most risk of HIV-related OIs and tumours, but some may not have significant symptoms or signs.

Whilst different HIV-associated conditions appear to correlate loosely with different CD4 counts (see table, below) there is excellent evidence that patients who start treatment at a CD4 count above 500 cells/μl, in comparison with below 500, are less likely to develop any serious AIDS or non-AIDS associated events.

6. Viral load

This is a measure of the amount of HIV in the blood, determined using a PCR test, and reflects rates of viral replication. Viral load can range from undetectable (defined as the sensitivity of the test – currently less than 20–50 copies of viral genome/ml of blood, depending on the assay) to over a million copies/ml. Numbers of copies/ml are expressed in a log

How CD4 counts correlate with HIV-related problems			
CD4 count cells/µl	Risk of opportunistic infection	Risk of HIV-associated tumours	Direct HIV effects
500 and below	Little risk	Hodgkin's disease Cervical cancer	
400 and below	Bacterial skin infections Recurrent bacterial chest infections Tuberculosis (TB) Oropharyngeal candida Fungal infections (skin, feet, nails) Seborrhoeic dermatitis		Lymphadenopathy Sweats
350 and below	Oral hairy leukoplakia Shingles *Pneumocystis* pneumonia Persistent herpes simplex infections	Non-Hodgkin's lymphoma	Weight loss
200 and below	Oesophageal candida Histoplasmosis Cryptococcal meningitis Cerebral toxoplasmosis Cryptosporidiosis	Kaposi's sarcoma	Diarrhoea Wasting
100 and below	Cytomegalovirus infections *Mycobacterium avium intracellulare*	Primary cerebral lymphoma	Dementia

Reproduced with permission from e-GP: e-Learning for General Practice (www.e-GP.org) ©Royal College of General Practitioners 2010.
Opportunistic infection column adapted from: Leake-Date H & Fisher M HIV Infection. In: Whittlesea C & Walker R (eds) (2007) *Clinical Pharmacy and Therapeutics 4th Edition*. Oxford: Churchill Livingstone.

scale (eg 10^6 copies/ml). The degree of viral replication is linked to the rate of CD4 decline and hence disease progression.

The viral load will fall if ART is acting effectively and the aim is to achieve viral suppression (generally taken as an undetectable viral load). A viral load which fails to fall, or which rises, in a patient on ART can indicate a range of problems. For example the patient may not be adhering to their regimen, there may be resistance of the virus to one or more antiretroviral drugs or blood levels of ART may be sub-therapeutic due to interaction with another medication. Resistance is commonly a consequence of episodes of non-adherence.

7. How the CD4 count and viral load interrelate

A high viral load predicts a more rapid CD4 decline. The CD4 count of those not taking ART and who have a high viral load is likely to fall more rapidly than that of those with a lower viral load (see figure 5). When the viral load is effectively suppressed by ART, CD4 counts recover with a lower risk of developing OIs, tumours and other complications.

Figure 5 | Association between virological, immunological and clinical events, and time course of HIV infection in an untreated individual

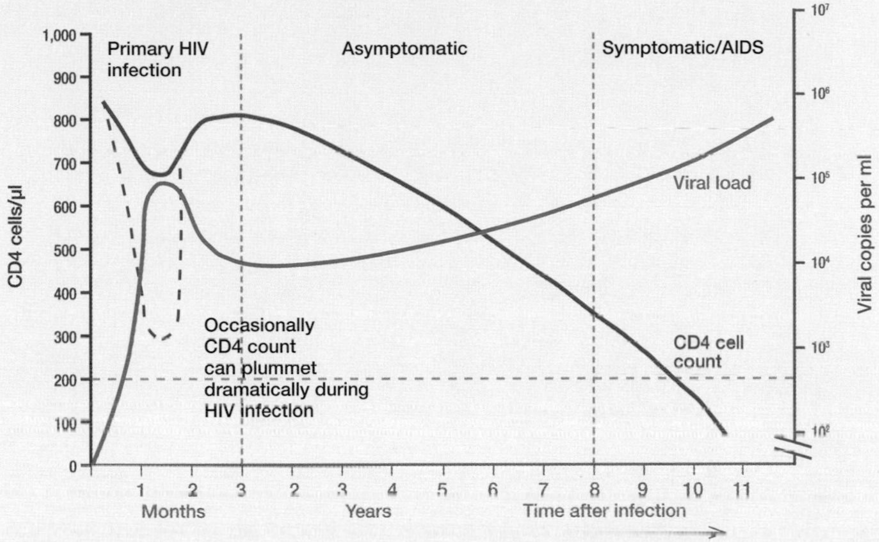

Reproduced with permission from e-GP: e-Learning for General Practice (www.e-GP.org) © Royal College of General Practitioners 2010

Antiretroviral therapy (ART)

For more on ART and side effects see pages 76–80

ART limits HIV replication with the aim of reducing viral load to undetectable levels. HIV mutates as it replicates and if drugs are used singly resistance rapidly develops. Therefore, drugs are most often used in combinations of three or more. Adherence to drug regimens is essential to prevent resistance.

ART has had an enormous impact on morbidity and mortality from HIV disease in the UK (see figure 1). ART is given not only to protect the health of patients but also to prevent transmission of the virus. The CD4 count at which ART is recommended has risen steadily over the years in the light of the findings of large studies, and UK guidelines now recommend that all HIV infected individuals are started on ART, irrespective of CD4 count. The lower the CD4 count the greater the benefits of ART.

This section gives a brief overview of the current specialist management of HIV. New drugs and strategies are continually being developed, although many patients will be successfully managed on one or two standard drug regimens.

For aspects of management that may be encountered by the GP, see the guide to managing HIV-related problems on pages 100–104.

Antiretroviral drugs are classified into five groups, according to where and how they act in the replication cycle of the virus. They are:
- nucleoside (or nucleotide) reverse transcriptase inhibitors (NRTIs)
- non-nucleoside reverse transcriptase inhibitors (NNRTIs)
- protease inhibitors (PIs)
- integrase inhibitors (IIs)
- entry inhibitors (EIs).

The effectiveness of ART is monitored by measuring viral load (see page 17). In the individual patient with an unsuppressed viral load, the strains of virus can also be tested for drug resistance mutations to help determine the best combination of antiretroviral drugs to use.

After ART has started, drugs may be changed according to any side effects experienced. These can include serious conditions such as hyperlipidaemia or chronic kidney impairment.

HIV prevention in the UK

At a strategic level, efforts to promote sexual health target those in groups associated with a high risk of HIV. It is sensible, for example, to prioritise interventions supporting safer sex with gay men, or projects working on knowledge of HIV and transmission risks among African communities. However, when a patient from one of these groups consults, those working in primary care should make no assumptions about risk. Each individual's risk needs to be assessed. For more on assessing risk, see page 48.

For more detailed information on sexual history-taking, risk assessment and sexual health promotion, see eLearning for Healthcare *eGP* – GP Curriculum sessions 3.08_01 to 08

1. Promoting safer sexual practices
Penetrative sex
Condom use significantly reduces sexually transmitted infections (STIs) and HIV transmission from both vaginal and anal sex. Condoms must be used both correctly and consistently to be effective. Condoms should be worn before penetration, and water-based or silicone-based lubricants should be used. Oil-based lubricants degrade latex. Condom failure is more often a function of inadequate lubrication and incorrect fitting than condom thickness. Ongoing inconsistent use of condoms may be associated with drug or alcohol problems – an assessment should be made.

Oral sex
The risk of HIV transmission through oral sex is very, very low; the combination of oral disease (ulceration, gingivitis) in the HIV-negative person and a very high viral load (such as in primary HIV infection) might

make transmission more likely. For a very small number of individuals this is the only risk factor in acquiring HIV infection. Avoiding ejaculation in the mouth is thought to decrease risk.

2. Preventing mother-to-child transmission

With appropriate interventions the transmission rate of HIV from mother to baby (vertical transmission) can be reduced to under 1 per cent. Achieving this depends on detecting HIV before pregnancy, or, failing that, in early pregnancy, when the chances of achieving viral suppression by the time of delivery are greatest.

See British HIV Association guidelines for the management of HIV infection in pregnant women 2012 (interim review May 2014)

Interventions to prevent vertical transmission include:
- ART in pregnancy
- ART at delivery plus a short course for the baby
- vaginal delivery for women on ART with an undetectable viral load; elective caesarian section for others
- avoidance of breastfeeding (breastfeeding advice differs in low income countries).

The ideal time to detect HIV infection is before the woman becomes pregnant. Offering HIV tests routinely to women using contraception – alongside tests for rubella immunity and haemoglobinopathy screens – is good practice, particularly in high prevalence areas. Add testing for viral hepatitis (B and C) if the woman is from a high prevalence country for these.

Remember that women may need to be offered further HIV tests if there has been a further risk of infection.

See Public Health England (2016) Infectious Diseases in Pregnancy Screening Programme Standards

Once pregnant, all women should be offered screening for hepatitis B and C, HIV, rubella susceptibility and syphilis as an integral part of their antenatal care.

3. Preventing transmission among injecting drug users

Preventing injecting drug use through education and information strategies is one approach. For those already injecting drugs, there are:

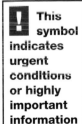

This symbol indicates urgent conditions or highly important information

- services that support people trying to quit and that prescribe safer substitutes such as methadone or buprenorphine
- services to support safer injecting practices. Needle exchanges are available in the community where drug users can exchange used needles and syringes for new replacements on an anonymous basis.

Injecting drugs or 'slamming' is an increasing practice amongst people engaging in 'chemsex' (predominantly gay men), and several sexual health services now provide 'slamming packs' containing injecting equipment and sharps disposal.

4. Reducing onward transmission from people with diagnosed HIV

See British HIV Association (BHIVA) and Expert Advisory Group on AIDS (EAGA) *Position statement on the use of antiretroviral therapy to reduce HIV transmission.* September 2014

The risks of transmission of HIV when people on ART are fully virally suppressed (ie with undetectable viral load) are massively reduced (ie by over 90 per cent). Two studies have demonstrated zero transmissions between couples where one is HIV-negative and the other is HIV-positive with an undetectable virus on ART. Thus full adherence to ART regimens should be supported, and problems with adherence or side effects addressed promptly.

People with diagnosed HIV infection should also be supported to follow safer sex and safer drug use practices as described above. For more on sexual and reproductive health issues for people with diagnosed HIV, see Section 3, pages 66–69.

5. Providing post-exposure prophylaxis (PEP): an emergency

For PEP following occupational exposure see page 94

PEP is the emergency use of ART to prevent infection when a person has been exposed to a known or high risk of HIV transmission. The aim is to give ART as soon as possible after exposure (ideally well within 24 hours, to a maximum of 72 hours). The exact choice of drug combination requires expert guidance and may involve more drugs at higher doses than 'normal' ART. The medication, usually taken for four weeks, can therefore have significant side effects and some people are unable to continue working while taking it.

PEP may be appropriate:

- following occupational exposure – see page 93 for management of needlestick injuries and PEP
- when an uninfected individual has had sex without a condom with a sexual partner known to have HIV or following sexual assault – see page 87 for post-exposure prophylaxis following sexual exposure (PEPSE).

In most situations PEP is no longer recommended if the HIV-positive partner is confirmed to have an undetectable viral load on ART. HIV specialists will be able to give urgent advice, and Accident and Emergency Departments generally have protocols to deal with PEP.

6. Pre-exposure prophylaxis (PrEP)

Giving ART to those at ongoing high risk of acquiring HIV has been demonstrated to be dramatically effective at preventing acquisition of the virus in higher risk men who have sex with men. Two separate studies found (identical) reductions in new infections of 86 per cent. This intervention is not currently commissioned on the NHS, although some people are obtaining PrEP medication privately, with or without NHS clinical advice and management. This could be a very significant finding when taking a medication history, posing a risk of drug interactions.

7. Screening blood and treating blood products

All blood donations in the UK have routinely been screened for HIV since 1985, and now tests include either PCR or antigen tests, alongside those for antibodies. All blood products in the UK are heat-treated to destroy HIV and other blood-borne viruses.

8. Immunisation

There is little prospect for an effective vaccine against HIV in the near future.

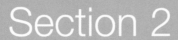

Section 2

How to diagnose HIV in primary care

IN THIS SECTION

How to diagnose HIV in primary care

People who are unaware that they have HIV are attending primary care. Which symptoms and conditions may be clues to HIV infection? How should HIV testing be approached in primary care?

Opportunities to diagnose HIV in primary care

There are two circumstances which provide valuable opportunities to diagnose HIV infection in primary care:

- when the patient presents with symptoms or medical conditions possibly associated with HIV – this is discussed in the first part of this section

See the *UK National Guidelines for HIV Testing 2008*

- offering an HIV test to an asymptomatic patient because they are or may be at risk of HIV infection – this is included in the second part of this section.

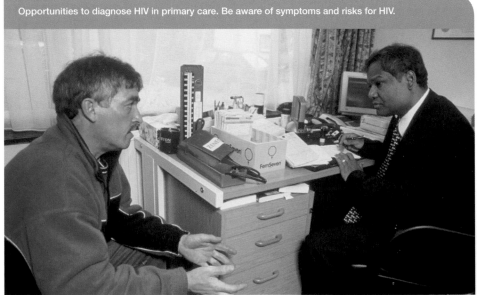

Opportunities to diagnose HIV in primary care. Be aware of symptoms and risks for HIV.

Talking to patients about HIV

This may be challenging to the clinician, especially if raising the subject with someone who is not expecting it. In this section we suggest verbal strategies that may be used in a variety of clinical situations. These are indicated in the speech bubbles on pages 51–53.

There are three important principles

Be open with the patient about the clinical reasoning behind your questions

A patient with a skin rash who is suddenly asked 'Can I ask if you are gay?' will wonder what the doctor is up to and, if he is gay, whether it is wise to answer honestly. If the doctor first lays out the clinical grounds for asking the question, the patient may be better prepared to give a full history. There are examples of how to do this later in the booklet.

Be non-judgemental

It is advisable to be direct but sensitive in your questioning. The more accessible and understanding you appear, the more trusting the patient will be, and the more accurate the replies. If the patient perceives the clinician to be disapproving or judgemental, they will be more likely to withhold information and may not return for future care and follow-up.

Ensure your service is (and is seen to be) confidential

Patients may have concerns about confidentiality, in primary care in particular. This may inhibit open discussion of personal issues. Ensure your practice develops a confidentiality policy and implements it through training and induction. Let your patients know that the policy is in place by displaying a confidentiality statement.

For practice policies and systems see page 91

The clinical diagnosis of HIV

There is evidence that a significant proportion of people who present late with HIV infection have been in contact with doctors in preceding years with symptoms which, in retrospect, were related to HIV. Late diagnosis of HIV infection contributes substantially to morbidity and mortality. More advanced disease leaves people vulnerable to overwhelming infection until their CD4 count has risen in response to treatment. Delay in diagnosis also increases the likelihood of onward transmission.

The clinical diagnosis of HIV-related conditions in primary care is not always easy. Many problems associated with HIV are commonly seen in people without HIV infection, for example, seborrhoeic dermatitis, shingles, folliculitis or a glandular fever-like illness. It barely seems feasible to consider HIV first – and then to raise it – whenever common conditions such as these present in the surgery.

Nevertheless, the GP is familiar with the concept of considering rare but serious conditions when extremely common symptoms present. We make quick assessments to answer questions such as 'Could this febrile child have meningitis?' or 'Could this headache be due to a brain tumour?' In this section we try to give the GP a realistic and pragmatic approach to improving their chances of detecting HIV infection.

There are two main clinical opportunities for diagnosing symptomatic HIV infection in primary care:
- primary HIV infection
- conditions associated with longstanding HIV infection.
  These are dealt with in turn.

Primary HIV infection

Primary HIV infection (PHI – also known as seroconversion illness) occurs soon after infection – usually between 10 days and six weeks. Symptoms develop in over 60 per cent of people at this stage. They may be mild and non-specific, but can also be marked and precipitate a consultation with the GP and, occasionally, hospital admission. Even a very HIV-aware doctor is likely to miss some patients with PHI.

> **IMPORTANT!**
> An HIV test is likely to be positive in primary infection, but the risk of a false negative is higher (see page 16). If in doubt, re-test in a week.

Primary HIV infection. A blotchy rash on the trunk is sometimes present two to six weeks after infection with HIV.

NICK BEECHING

Diagnosis of primary HIV infection is valuable because:
- the next opportunity for diagnosis may be at a late stage of disease progression, and so the prognosis for the patient is likely to be much worse
- identifying the infection may protect others from becoming infected
- ART is now recommended for patients with PHI: there is evidence that treatment may be particularly protective at this stage.

Symptoms and signs of PHI
The patient may have none, some or all of these:
- fever

- sore throat
- maculopapular rash on the trunk
- malaise/lethargy
- arthralgia and myalgia
- lymphadenopathy
- oral, genital or perianal ulcers.

Other features that are less commonly present include:
- headache or meningism
- diarrhoea
- weight loss.

IMPORTANT!
Thinking glandular fever?

Two recent studies have shown an HIV prevalence of 3.9 per cent and 1.3 per cent in patients presenting with glandular fever type symptoms. If, as the clinician, you find yourself asking for blood tests to exclude glandular fever, remember to consider primary HIV infection

The CD4 count may drop sharply at this stage of HIV infection, although will usually recover, and so acute conditions associated with immunosuppression may also occur, including:
- oral candidiasis
- shingles
- other conditions associated with immunodeficiency (see pages 31–41).

What to do if you suspect primary HIV infection
Nothing is going to make this an easy consultation. As the symptoms can resolve within three weeks, you will need to act quickly if you think the patient has PHI.

1. Take a history and conduct an examination to look for further evidence of PHI. Has the person had a rash? Or sores or ulcers in the mouth or genital area? (Even if the person has PHI, there may be no additional features).

2. If you remain concerned, raise it with the patient. "Illnesses like this are usually caused by viruses, for example the glandular fever or flu virus. Some quite rare viruses can also be a cause, and it is important that I don't miss them if they occur. I don't know if you are at risk, but HIV is one of these." To move on to a risk assessment of the last 12 weeks: "Could I ask you a few questions to see if you could be at risk?"

3. If the patient has clinical features of PHI, or if they have an identified risk, then recommend the test and offer safer sex advice at this point. The result will be back in about a week so make an appointment for them to attend.

4. If the result is positive, arrange referral to HIV specialist services. If negative, retest (one week after the first test), reiterating the safer sex advice.

For more on assessing risk see page 48

5. If the second result is negative, this is highly likely to exclude PHI.

case study

A man with a flu-like illness

Ian, a 28-year-old white British male, had been registered with the practice two years, but had only attended once before, for smoking cessation advice. He attended his GP saying he had flu and felt dreadful. He said he was exhausted and was now in the eighth day of his illness. He had a sore throat, ached all over and felt feverish.

The GP considered it might be glandular fever, or possibly HIV. First, she asked Ian about rashes (he had none) and oral and genital ulceration. Ian said he had mouth ulcers. On examination the GP could see three.

After discussing glandular fever, the GP raised the subject of HIV and explained that very rarely an illness like this might be caused in the early weeks of HIV infection. The GP took a partner history and established that Ian lived with his male partner, a relationship of six years. Ian indicated that he felt that his relationship was mutually monogamous. There was no history of drug use.

The discussion appeared to make Ian anxious, so the GP said: 'On the basis of what you have told me your illness is unlikely to be primary HIV infection.' She asked Ian if he would be interested in having an HIV test 'in any case' and he said he would consider it. Ian returned within a week and explained that he had had unprotected sex five weeks before with a new partner he had met in a club. He had now discussed the situation fully with his partner at home, and had decided to have a test. She took a sample

> The GP considered it might be glandular fever or possibly HIV. First, she asked Ian about rashes (he had none) and oral and genital ulceration. Ian said he had mouth ulcers. On examination the GP could see three.

and the test was found to be HIV p24 antigen positive, but antibody negative, confirming primary HIV infection. Ian was initially distressed and overwhelmed by feelings of guilt. Hospital follow-up was arranged.

Ian's long-term partner, Will, was also registered with the practice. The couple were seen together and it was established that they had had one episode of unprotected sex between the time Ian had contracted the infection and the time he initially saw the GP. Then they hadn't had sex until some time after HIV infection was confirmed. Will tested negative both initially and three months later. Six months after this the relationship had survived and the couple were continuing to practise safer sex. Ian was optimistic, had been started on ART and had returned to work. The couple told the GP that they felt that Will had been saved from getting HIV because she had been 'so on the ball'.

Learning points

- In many consultations, important aspects of the sexual history will not simply be volunteered: it is of value to ask directly.
- There are people in some groups (for example men who have sex with men, or people who sell sex) who may be much less likely to disclose relevant information.
- Strategies for sexual history taking that avoid assumptions and judgements will often help.
- Sexual partners of anyone diagnosed with HIV should be offered an HIV test as routine.

Clinical indicator conditions associated with untreated HIV infection

Problems associated with HIV infection may be subtle and insidious, and patients may recover and be well for some time before encountering another problem. Subtle symptoms may mask serious illness, and conditions GPs may have been trained to think were harmless may indicate HIV disease.

IMPORTANT!

Don't miss urgent or life-threatening conditions. Don't miss PCP!

Memorise the conditions in this section that are highlighted as urgent by the symbol above.

Most serious problems usually occur at very low CD4 counts (below 100 cells/µl) so other clinical clues to immunosuppression are likely to be present.

Pneumocystis pneumonia (PCP) is an exception to this rule as it tends to occur at higher CD4 counts (below 200). It may be the first HIV-related problem for which the patient seeks advice. The prognosis correlates directly with how early or late the infection is identified and treated: PCP can kill if diagnosed too late.

When you encounter any of the conditions given in this section, allow the thought of HIV to go through your mind. The stakes are high for these patients – HIV diagnosis at this presentation may be life-saving. The possibility of immunosuppression is especially important to explore if:

- the patient has had more than one of the conditions listed below in the preceding two or three years; or the patient has had an unusually severe or difficult to treat form of any of the conditions listed below.

There are many examples of patients being referred to secondary care with these symptoms without being tested for HIV. This delays diagnosis and wastes time and money with patients attending outpatient clinics – such as medical, gastro, dermatology, ENT, gynaecology and others – for expensive (and frequently irrelevant) investigations. It may also put others at risk of acquiring HIV.

Guidance for assessing problems that may be HIV-related

- **Enquire** about weight loss, sweats, diarrhoea
- **Examine** the patient for other signs of immunosuppression (mouth, skin and nodes)
- **Review** the records for evidence of HIV-associated problems (see list on pages 32–40)
- **Discuss** the possibility of HIV with the patient to consider their risk
- **Decide** on priorities: is urgent assessment by a specialist required or can an HIV test be offered?

Mouth, skin and nodes see pages 37–39

Think HIV and be prepared to offer the test – don't assume someone else will do it!

For table of clinical indicator conditions see page 105

A number of conditions are commoner in those who have HIV infection: they are associated with greater or lesser degrees of immunosuppression. However, many of these 'indicator conditions' also arise frequently in those uninfected with HIV. If a GP encounters, or diagnoses, any of these conditions they should, in general, offer an HIV test; or at the very least think it through.

1. Respiratory conditions

Cough, sweats, shortness of breath and weight loss may be caused by several opportunistic infections, including community-acquired bacterial infections such as pneumonia. *Pneumocystis* pneumonia (PCP) is an important infection but may be insidious and so easier to miss. TB is also important. Occasionally, lymphomas or Kaposi's sarcoma may affect the lungs in HIV-infected patients.

PCP
This is a life-threatening infection with symptoms which often have an insidious onset progressing over several weeks. Arguably, PCP is the single most dangerous trap for the unwary GP as it may be the first HIV-related clinical problem the patient has. The prognosis correlates directly with how early or late the infection is identified and treated: PCP can kill if diagnosed late.

Symptoms
- a persistent dry cough of a few weeks' duration
- increasing shortness of breath or decreasing exercise tolerance (clinicians should ask because patients may not mention it)
- difficulty in taking a full breath (this reflects loss of elasticity of the lung tissue)
- fever (in most but not all).

Assessment
The chest is often clear on auscultation – especially in early stages. Fine crackles may be heard. Pulse oximetry may reveal a fall in oxygen saturation after the patient is asked to, for example, walk up and down stairs. Chest X-rays may reveal little and can lead to delay. The GP may be thinking of asthma, an atypical chest infection or anxiety. If PCP is a possibility, look for evidence of HIV: see the guidance on assessment above and also boxed information on page 41.

Management/referral
Refer the patient urgently if you are concerned they may have PCP, which can only be diagnosed by hospital-based tests such as induced sputum

and bronchoscopy. An HIV test may cause inappropriate delay.

This condition is also important to detect in any patient known to have HIV, even if they are on medication to prevent this. PCP is most often seen in those with CD4 counts of less than 200 cells/μl, but about 10 per cent have a CD4 above 200 cells/μl, so a CD4 at this level should not be a reason to exclude PCP.

TB and atypical mycobacterial disease

TB is an important and common presenting problem in HIV-infected patients in the UK. It can occur at CD4 counts above 200. People with HIV are more likely to develop symptoms and/or systemic infection with TB than those without HIV.

Atypical mycobacterial disease (*Mycobacterium avium intracellulare*) is a less common complication, associated with late-stage HIV infection.

> See case study
> page 43

Symptoms

The patient may have a cough, fever, sweats, shortness of breath, weight loss or haemoptysis. They may have associated large, asymmetrical nodes.

Mycobacterium avium intracellulare may present with systemic symptoms and chest symptoms may or may not be present. Abnormal liver function tests and anaemia may be found.

> Guidelines recommend Anyone diagnosed with TB should be tested for HIV.

Assessment

As for TB in the HIV-negative (eg chest X-ray), but look for evidence of HIV: see guidance on assessment on page 31 and also boxed information on page 41. *Mycobacterium avium intracellulare* is very unlikely in a patient without several clinical pointers to HIV disease because it occurs at very low CD4 counts.

Management/referral

Urgent outpatient or inpatient referral will be required, although an HIV test could also be arranged and may save time if the patient is not too unwell.

> For guidance on assessment see box on page 31

Community-acquired chest infections

Chest infections which respond to the antibiotics usually employed in community settings are commoner in immunosuppressed patients.

> Guidelines recommend Anyone with bacterial pneumonia should be offered an HIV test.

Assessment

Look for evidence of HIV: see guidance on assessment on page 31, and also boxed information on page 41.

Management/referral

As usual for chest infections, but offer an HIV test if appropriate.

2. Conditions causing neurological and visual symptoms

A great variety of intracranial or peripheral neurological problems may occur in relation to HIV infection. Symptoms and signs include:

- headache, neck stiffness or photophobia
- focal neurological signs suggesting intracranial space occupying lesion (for example, lymphoma)
- peripheral neuropathy (especially sensory change or loss)
- confusion, memory loss, or disinhibition
- fits.

Cryptococcal meningitis
This may present with headaches without the classical symptoms or signs of meningism.

Assessment
Apart from a neurological assessment and general examination, look for evidence of HIV. See guidance on assessment on page 31.

Management/referral
The patient will need to be referred urgently. An HIV test may cause inappropriate delay if the patient is very unwell.

Toxoplasmosis
This may present with headaches, fever and focal neurological signs which may be progressive.

Assessment
Apart from a neurological assessment and general examination, look for evidence of HIV. See guidance on assessment on page 31.

Management/referral
The patient will need to be referred urgently. Waiting for an HIV test may cause inappropriate delay if the diagnosis is suspected.

Cerebral lymphoma
This may present with headaches, fever and focal neurological signs which may be progressive.

Assessment
Apart from a neurological assessment and general examination, look for evidence of HIV. See guidance on assessment on page 31.

Management/referral

The patient will need to be referred urgently. Waiting for an HIV test may cause inappropriate delay if the diagnosis is suspected.

Cytomegalovirus (CMV) infection of the retina

CMV infection of the retina causes blindness and can be treated, but earlier diagnosis improves the prognosis. It is mostly found in those who have CD4 counts below 100 cells/µl.

The patient may have:

- floaters
- reduced vision
- scotomas.

> **For CD4 counts see page 17**

Assessment

Changes may be visible on fundoscopy, but the absence of changes should not alter management. Look for evidence of HIV: see guidance on assessment on page 31. CMV retinitis is very unlikely in a patient without several clinical pointers to HIV disease, because it occurs at very low CD4 counts.

> **For guidance on assessment see box on page 31**

Management/referral

The patient will need to be referred urgently to ophthalmology. Waiting for the result of an HIV test may cause inappropriate delay if the patient is very unwell.

> **Guidelines recommend Anyone with suspected CMV or with any unexplained retinopathy should be offered an HIV test.**

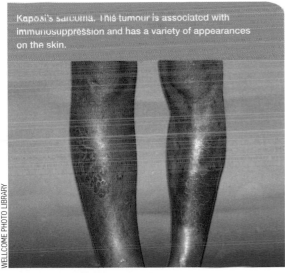

Kaposi's sarcoma. This tumour is associated with immunosuppression and has a variety of appearances on the skin.

WELLCOME PHOTO LIBRARY

> Guidelines recommend **Anyone diagnosed with lymphoma should routinely be offered an HIV test.**

3. Tumours associated with HIV

Lymphoma

Both non-Hodgkin and Hodgkin lymphoma are associated with HIV. They may cause lymphadenopathy, fevers, night sweats and abdominal masses. They may be cerebral (see neurological problems, page 34).

Assessment

Look for evidence of HIV. See guidance on assessment on page 31.

Management/referral

As for any suspected cancer.

Cervical carcinoma and other HPV-associated cancers

Cervical cancer may cause vaginal bleeding or discharge. Cytological abnormalities may also be a marker for underlying HIV infection and so the offer of an HIV test is good practice.

Other human papilloma virus (HPV)-associated cancers are also commoner including anal, vulval, vaginal and some head and neck cancers.

Assessment and management/referral

As normal for suspected cancer. Offer an HIV test if appropriate.

Kaposi's sarcoma (KS)

These tumours may occur in a variety of places. They most commonly appear as dark purple or brown intradermal lumps that sometimes look like bruises (but feel harder). KS may also be found in the mouth. Infiltration of the lungs or gut is rare but can be very serious, the latter causing gastrointestinal (GI) bleeding.

Kaposi's sarcoma. This tumour may also rarely affect the gut.

Assessment and management/referral

Conduct an HIV test. Refer to an HIV specialist. May require urgent medical admission if there is evidence of lung or gut involvement.

Other cancers

A number of other cancers are also HIV-associated including lung, renal, colorectal and liver cancer (the latter associated with viral hepatitis co-infection). Melanomas, seminomas and Castleman's disease are also commoner.

Guidelines recommend Anyone with mononucleosis-like syndrome, PUO (pyrexia of unknown origin), weight loss of >10kg or lymphadenopathy of unknown cause should be offered an HIV test.

4. Constitutional symptoms associated with HIV

Constitutional symptoms may be caused by HIV itself, or by a related opportunistic infection (such as TB) or tumour (such as a lymphoma). Symptoms include:

- flu-like symptoms (see page 28)
- fever
- weight loss
- sweats
- lymphadenopathy (HIV is particularly likely if this persists in excess of three months, in two or more extra-inguinal sites and in the absence of any other cause).

See case study page 44

Assessment
Look for evidence of HIV, see guidance on page 31.

Management/referral
Urgent assessment is sometimes appropriate. For outpatient referrals arrange an HIV test beforehand to ensure that the appropriate clinic is identified and inform them of the result. For inpatient referrals, highlight the need for HIV testing in the referral letter.

For guidance on assessment see box on page 31

5. Skin conditions

Look out for common skin conditions that are particularly severe or hard to treat. Review the records for other evidence of HIV infection. Examples include:

See case study page 45

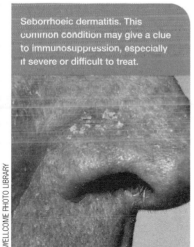

Seborrhoeic dermatitis. This common condition may give a clue to immunosuppression, especially if severe or difficult to treat.

- **fungal infections**, such as tinea cruris, tinea pedis, pityriasis versicolor
- **viral infections**, such as shingles (especially if more than one dermatome is affected), *Molluscum contagiosum*, warts and herpes simplex
- **bacterial infections**, such as impetigo, folliculitis
- **Kaposi's sarcoma** (see above for description)
- **other skin conditions**, such as seborrhoeic dermatitis and psoriasis.

Assessment
Look for evidence of HIV. See guidance on assessment on page 31, and also boxed information on page 41.

Management/referral
As usual, and arrange an HIV test if appropriate.

6. Conditions affecting the mouth

Guidelines recommend Anyone with oral candidiasis and/or oral hairy leukoplakia should be offered an HIV test.

Immunosuppression can lead to a number of conditions affecting the mouth and examination of the mouth is key in assessment as some of the conditions may be asymptomatic. Examples include:

- **oral candidiasis** (thrush): not just a coated tongue, but thick white plaques on the buccal mucosa that could be scraped off with a tongue depressor. Oral candida can also have a red, fleshy appearance with fewer – or no – plaques and in this case can be harder to diagnose. Swabs are of little diagnostic value because of high carriage rates. Florid oral thrush should always lead to a consideration of whether the patient could be immunosuppressed.
- **aphthous ulceration**
- **oral hairy leukoplakia**: causing whitish corrugations, typically on the side of the tongue. They cannot be scraped off. It is usually asymptomatic, but is pathognomic of immunosuppression. It is useful to look for this if you suspect a patient may have HIV disease (see photo on page 39)
- **Kaposi's sarcoma**: purple tumour, characteristically on the palate
- **gingivitis**
- **dental abscesses**.

Assessment
Look for evidence of HIV: see guidance on assessment on page 31, and also boxed information on page 41.

Management/referral
As usual and arrange an HIV test if appropriate.

7. Conditions affecting the upper and lower GI tract

Guidelines recommend Anyone with chronic diarrhoea or oral/ oesophageal candidiasis should be offered an HIV test.

Significant conditions include:
- **oesophageal candidiasis**: the patient presents with dysphagia suggestive of an oesophageal problem, but is highly likely to have concurrent oral thrush
- **diarrhoea** – persistent mild, or severe acute. There may be virtually any – or commonly no – causative organism found.

Assessment
Look for evidence of HIV.

Management/referral
As usual and arrange an HIV test if appropriate.

For guidance on assessment see box on page 31

Left to right:
1. Oral candida. This condition is an important indicator of immunosuppression.
2. Oral hairy leukoplakia. Pathognomic of immunosuppression.
3. Palatal Kaposi's sarcoma. This tumour gives another reason for careful examination of the mouth when looking for evidence of HIV.

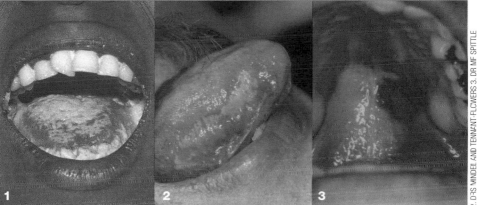

1. VAN DEN HOMBERGH/P.3H/WELLCOME PHOTO LIBRARY

2. D3S MINDEL AND TENNANT-FLOWERS 3. DR MF SPITTLE

8. Genital problems

> Guidelines recommend **Anyone diagnosed with an STI should be routinely tested for HIV.**

Severe or difficult to treat genital candida may be a clue to immunosuppression, and tests for both diabetes and HIV should be considered. Sexually transmitted infections (STIs) such as genital herpes or genital warts may be more severe in the immunosuppressed patient. The diagnosis of any STI should lead to the offer of an HIV test.

See case study page 40

Assessment
Look for evidence of HIV: see guidance on assessment on page 31, and also boxed information on page 41.

Management/referral
As usual and arrange an HIV test if appropriate.

See also cervical cancer page 36

9. Haematological problems

Changes found on routine full blood counts may give a clue to immunosuppression. They may be severe enough to require urgent action, but are often subtle, with few symptoms. Examples include anaemia, neutropenia, lymphopenia, thrombocytopenia and diffuse hypergammaglobulinaemia.

> Guidelines recommend
> **Offering an HIV test to anyone with:**
> • neutropenia
> • anaemia
> • thrombocytopenia
> • any other unexplained blood dyscrasia.

Assessment

Look for evidence of HIV: see guidance on assessment on page 31, and also boxed information below.

Management/referral

As usual and arrange an HIV test if appropriate.

10. Viral hepatitis

Viral hepatitis may be associated with HIV. In the UK, most hepatitis B is due to being born or raised in a country with a high prevalence (by transmission from the mother or in early childhood). Most hepatitis C is due to injecting practices or unsafe treatment overseas (notably, Egypt). However, both hepatitis B and hepatitis C are also transmitted within the UK, particularly amongst men who have sex with men who have sexual and/or drug-taking risks including use of drugs as sexual stimulants ('chemsex').

It is very important that every patient with hepatitis B is tested for HIV. This is because antiviral monotherapy is used for hepatitis B and this may lead to resistance if HIV is present.

While co-infection with hepatitis B and HIV is common, there is a great deal more undiagnosed viral hepatitis in the UK than undiagnosed HIV. Tests for all these infections can stem from the same risk assessment questions (country of origin, injecting practices of any kind, sexual history).

> **IMPORTANT!**
> **Test for HIV before treating hepatitis B**
>
> It is essential to test anyone diagnosed with hepatitis B for HIV. Antiviral monotherapy to treat hepatitis B in an individual with undiagnosed HIV may result in HIV drug resistance.

What to do if you suspect HIV infection may underlie the presenting problem

If the problem is clinically minor (seborrhoeic dermatitis in a patient who had multidermatomal shingles two months ago), it may be reasonable to arrange an early review of the patient in order to give yourself time to collect your thoughts. But don't risk losing patients to follow-up. Remember that resolution of the presenting problem does not mean that HIV has been ruled out.

- **Enquire** about weight loss, sweats, diarrhoea.
- **Examine** the patient for other signs of immunosuppression (mouth, skin and nodes, see pages 37–39).
- **Review** the records for evidence of HIV-associated problems in the last three years (see list, pages 32–40).
- **Discuss** the possibility of HIV with the patient to consider their risk.

For many GPs raising the subject of HIV with the patient is difficult. For more details on risk assessment, see pages 48–49 and for suggested phrases for raising the question of an HIV test, see pages 51–53.

- **Decide on priorities**: is urgent assessment by a specialist required or can an HIV test be offered?

For more on risk assessment see pages 48–49

If the clinical picture is strongly suggestive of HIV, an apparent absence of risk of infection should not deter you from offering a test.

Diagnosing HIV in children

In 2014 there were 928 children (aged under 18 years) living with diagnosed HIV infection in the UK. This is an aging cohort with an average age of around 13 years. Challenges facing these children include adherence and, for adolescents, sexual health.

Children may be diagnosed with HIV because they present with symptoms or because they are tested after their parents or siblings are found to be HIV-infected. If you know a parent has HIV, check that all children have been tested. A small subset of those HIV-infected at birth have stayed healthy until 20 years of age without treatment (or diagnosis) – therefore reassurance that a child or young person is healthy should <u>not</u> be taken as a reason not to test.

If an infant or child presents with symptoms or conditions that cause concern, do not let a belief that the mother is HIV-negative put you off considering HIV. Occasionally, a mother who tests negative at antenatal screening may acquire HIV later in the pregnancy and remain undiagnosed after her child is born.

Presenting conditions and indications for testing:

Infants most often present with failure to thrive, and/or pneumocystis pneumonia, CMV disease or HIV encephalopathy.

After the first year of life HIV testing should be considered, discussed and arranged with any of the following presentations:
- recurrent infections (eg of the ear, chest or skin or upper respiratory tract infections)
- severe manifestations of common childhood infections (eg severe chicken pox).
- severe pneumonia
- TB
- chronic painless swelling of the parotid glands
- chronic enlargement of the cervical gland
- any indicator condition in the adult list (see page 105)

Lymphoid interstitial pneumonitis is usually asymptomatic, but has a characteristic appearance on chest X-ray and can be difficult to distinguish from miliary TB. The appearance is due to infiltration of the lungs with nodules of inflammatory lymphocytes.

case study

Late diagnosis of HIV and tuberculosis

Jemi is a 26-year-old woman who came to the UK from Sierra Leone two years ago. She saw her GP with a six-week history of fevers, intermittent cough and cervical lymphadenopathy. Nine months previously she had attended her GP with fatigue and was found to have mild anaemia. Now she was prescribed penicillin V, which alleviated her symptoms for a few days. A week later she presented again with rigors, night sweats and weight loss. She was admitted to hospital for investigation of pyrexia of unknown origin with malaria at the top of the differential diagnosis.

She was found to have non-tender 'rubbery' lymphadenopathy in her axilliary, inguinal, supraclavicular and cervical areas. On admission she also had a fever of 30.1°C and a tachycardia. She was hypotensive, had 2–3cms hepatomegaly and otherwise no focal signs in her chest, abdomen or central nervous system.

She was treated with multiple antibiotics but did not improve. Following discussion with a member of the HIV team she reluctantly agreed to an HIV test, which was positive. She was eventually diagnosed with TB following sputum culture.

The history that emerged when she felt better was that she had been feeling 'ill' for at least six to eight weeks, and had had intermittent fevers (and some night sweats) for three months. She had been complaining of non-specific fatigue/malaise for at least eight or nine months, for which the full blood count had been the only investigation. She might not have agreed to an HIV test at that time, but an earlier diagnosis might have enabled her to avoid hospitalisation.

> She had been complaining of non-specific fatigue/malaise for at least eight or nine months, for which the full blood count had been the only investigation. She might not have agreed to an HIV test at that time, but an earlier diagnosis might have enabled her to avoid hospitalisation.

Learning points
- HIV testing is recommended for patients presenting with pyrexia of unknown origin and weight loss.
- HIV should be considered in people from areas of high HIV prevalence, regardless of their presentation.

case study

A delayed diagnosis

Ganesh is a 49-year-old divorced university lecturer. He attended his GP some months ago with diarrhoea and weight loss. Stool culture/microscopy revealed no apparent pathogen and there was little response to anti-diarrhoeal medication. He was referred to the local hospital where he was seen and placed on the waiting list for both upper GI endoscopy and a flexible sigmoidoscopy. This was performed four months after the original referral letter, his symptoms having continued and his overall weight loss being some 10 per cent of his original weight.

After the procedure he had to stay in hospital for two nights as he appeared to have developed an aspiration pneumonia. Broad-spectrum antibiotic treatment did very little and he was re-admitted four days later. Bronchoscopy confirmed a diagnosis of PCP, for which he was admitted and treated without further complication.

The only recorded social history was that he was divorced and smoked 20 cigarettes daily. He was not embarrassed to tell the doctors that he had sex with other men, but nobody had ever asked him. He was not surprised by the subsequent HIV diagnosis. His CD4 count was 49 cells/µl and he has done well since starting combination ART.

Learning points

- HIV testing is recommended for patients presenting with persistent unresolved diarrhoea and weight loss.
- If the symptoms could indicate HIV infection it is important to offer an HIV test even if a risk assessment has not been done, or no risk behaviour has been disclosed by the patient.

case study

A 'low-risk' man

Russell is a 33-year-old of UK origin who first presented to the practice nurse during a new patient medical following a house move. He lived with his girlfriend of eight years. At registration he complained of a rash on his face. This was red, dry and flaky and affected his forehead and his naso-labial folds. He was given a topical hydrocortisone/antifungal cream.

Twelve months later he returned to the practice and saw a locum GP following three days of non-specific abdominal pain and fever. He returned again to the practice after 10 days with a dry cough, fatigue and lethargy. He was given a broad-spectrum antibiotic but 14 days later was worse, and had developed a generalised maculopapular rash. The facial rash had returned, since he had run out of cream. He had lost 4kg of weight.

Frustrated at being off work for so long, he requested a referral to the local hospital where he was seen by a consultant physician three weeks later. Tests carried out by the GP in advance revealed a slight thrombocytopenia, mild elevation of his liver transaminases and a raised erythrocyte sedimentation rate (ESR). A chest X-ray was reported as normal. Russell was asked if he had ever injected drugs and stated that he had not done so. Serology for hepatitis B was negative. Physical examination by the hospital consultant revealed no abnormalities and an ultrasound of his liver was arranged.

Another three weeks passed, with no scan appointment arriving. Russell reported a worsening of his cough and extreme fatigue. He had marked dyspnoea on exertion. Two days later his girlfriend took him to casualty. By this time his dyspnoea had worsened, his weight loss continued and he had a dry cough. He was found to be tachypnoeic and hypoxic. His CXR showed patchy shadowing. The medical team felt he probably had *Pneumocystis* pneumonia (PCP). This was later confirmed on bronchoscopy. Russell tested positive for HIV and his CD4 count was only 10 cells/μl. Following the successful treatment of his PCP and initiation of ART, he returned to work and remains well.

> With no apparent risk factors to suggest a significant probability of HIV infection, and with such an insidious onset, the diagnosis eluded many practitioners until Russell was quite seriously ill.

With no apparent risk factors to suggest a significant probability of HIV infection, and with such an insidious onset, the diagnosis eluded many practitioners until Russell was quite seriously ill. It is probable that he acquired HIV through a sexual contact many years previously when he was travelling in Thailand and South East Asia in his student years.

Learning points

- Some people with HIV have no obvious risk factors for HIV infection.
- HIV infection can often exacerbate common skin conditions.
- Consider PCP in patients with recent onset dyspnoea or where atypical or severe respiratory infection is possible.
- Don't forget to ask about travel to areas of high HIV prevalence when taking a history.

case study

All STI diagnoses can signal risk

A 52-year-old woman of Egyptian origin, S, presented with genital warts. She had not been in a relationship for 18 months. She was otherwise well. An HIV test was offered as routine, although the GP was most concerned to exclude hepatitis C because of the high prevalence in Egypt. However it transpired that the patient had HIV – and not hepatitis C. A former partner, who had died under unclear circumstances, had come from a country with a high prevalence for HIV. S is taking ART, although depression has affected her adherence at times.

Learning points

- Every patient diagnosed with an STI, without exception, should be offered an HIV test.
- Testing for viral hepatitis is also clinically valuable as effective treatment is available.

case study

An older man

Mr L is a 76-year-old married British man of Indian origin. Having been well, he then developed unexplained anaemia, presenting with fatigue.

He was referred for urgent upper and lower GI endoscopy to exclude malignancy, and both proved normal. After this he developed diarrhoea, and some weight loss. He was referred back to gastroenterology, but further investigations revealed nothing.

His GP considered HIV but thought it unlikely. However due to the worrying symptoms he decided to discuss this with his patient. It turned out that Mr L had business interests in South Africa and frequently travelled there. He denied having sex with anyone apart from his wife of 37 years, but agreed to have an HIV test. This proved positive. Mr L responded very well to treatment, and his wife tested negative. She has been very supportive of him and they have remained together.

Learning points

- Do not make assumptions on the basis of age. New diagnosis is usually made in patients in their 30s and 40s, but of those diagnosed over 60 a significant proportion are diagnosed late: probably because of wrong assumptions.

HIV testing in primary care

Reducing the amount of undiagnosed HIV in the UK is a priority. Individuals who know they are infected with HIV have significant advantages over those who are infected but unaware of this. They will:

- benefit from current treatments resulting in an improved prognosis
- have information which may enable them to avoid passing on the virus
- become less infectious once on ART
- have the opportunity to reflect and plan ahead.

See the *UK National Guidelines for HIV Testing 2008*

1. The practicalities

What is the HIV test?

There are different types of HIV test. The most commonly used tests detect both HIV antibodies and antigens on a venous blood sample, and will usually become positive by 2 weeks after infection, but should be repeated at 4 weeks after risk if the first test is negative.

See page 28 for information on primary HIV infection

Antibody only tests (in general, rapid 'point of care' fingerprick or saliva tests) may miss early infection and are less suitable when primary HIV infection is being considered or if there have been risks in the preceding 4 weeks. If you have access to rapid tests, in this situation it may be appropriate to take an additional venous sample for a conventional HIV test.

For the types of HIV test including POCT see pages 15–17

All positive test results should be confirmed (the risks of a false positive are higher with rapid tests).

HIV testing and insurance reports

GPs should not allow insurance concerns to compromise patient care: if an HIV test is appropriate, it should be offered. The BMA website has guidance on confidentiality and health records, including medical information and insurance.

USEFUL INFO

The Association of British Insurers (ABI) states that insurers should only ask about positive, not negative, HIV tests. A *GP report insurance package* has been jointly produced by the ABI and British Medical Association, including a standard GP report form.

Laboratory support

The lab will need a clotted sample. Some smaller hospital laboratories only run HIV tests on certain days. Larger hospitals have several runs on a daily basis. Phone the lab to check:

- when HIV tests are processed
- when the results will be available
- what their procedure will be if they find an apparent positive.

Typically a lab will call when they find a positive result, and request a repeat sample.

Links with specialist HIV treatment centre(s)

The best time to find out about local HIV treatment centres and to establish links with them is before you have a patient who tests positive. This will ensure that clear referral pathways are in place, including details of who to contact if a patient needs to be seen urgently by a specialist.

Computer and paper systems to support HIV testing

See page 92 for discussion of systems and record keeping.

2. When should an HIV test be offered?

There are a number of circumstances in which it is appropriate to conduct an HIV test in primary care:

- patient request
- opportunistic testing – when an HIV test is offered to someone who might be at risk including anyone diagnosed with an STI (including chlamydia or genital warts, for example).
- diagnostic testing – when an HIV test is done because someone has an indicator condition, or symptoms or signs of HIV infection
- screening – for example antenatal screening. Population screening of newly registering patients in higher prevalence areas is recommended in UK guidelines and being implemented in some areas (definitions of high prevalence may change but it is currently greater than 2 diagnosed /1000 population aged 15 to 59).

If the test is offered on a routine or opt-out basis, evidence suggests it makes offering the test easier as it is perceived as non-judgemental and it is more likely to be accepted.

The patient who requests an HIV test

Patients requesting an HIV test will have a reason. After assessment, you may choose to be reassuring but avoid discouraging patients from testing and take care before declining to test.

> **IMPORTANT!**
> Any patient diagnosed with an STI should be offered an HIV test

> For the window period and different types of HIV test see pages 15–17

Patients may or may not be prepared to discuss their risks with you: however ensure the patient understands the significance of the window period and what constitutes risk. If doubts remain, arrange a second test at the appropriate time.

Occasionally anxiety (without any risk, or further risk, of infection) is at the root of repeated requests for HIV tests; in this case further testing is not indicated and the patient needs help to address their anxiety.

The patient may have an identified risk

As HIV infection may be asymptomatic for some time, the only hope of improving primary care detection rates in this group is if clinicians are willing and able to discuss risk of HIV and offer tests as appropriate. Risk of HIV can be identified by taking a routine travel, drug and sexual history for the purposes of health promotion.

The following should be offered a test if they have never been tested, or if they have been at risk since their last test. Those who:

- are from an area with a high prevalence of HIV (although risk should be discussed without pre-judgement as many people in this group may be at no risk)
- have a current or former sexual partner who is infected with HIV (particularly if they are not on ART, or taking it reliably), or from an area with a high prevalence of HIV or who was an injecting drug user
- are men who have had sex with other men
- are female sexual contacts of men who have sex with men
- have had multiple sexual partners
- have a history of sexually transmitted infection
- have a history of injecting drug use
- have been raped (although in an acute situation this is best managed by specialist services if the patient will attend)
- have had blood transfusions, transplants or other risk prone procedures in some low and middle income countries
- may have had an occupational exposure.

Careful condom use will have offered significant protection – this should be acknowledged, even if testing still goes ahead. Be ready to test anyone who requests an HIV test after their history has been taken, even if they have not indicated a specific risk to you.

> **IMPORTANT!**
> **Make sure all pregnant women are offered and recommended an HIV test. Interventions can reduce the risk of mother-to-child transmission from over 20 per cent to less than 1 per cent.**

The patient has symptoms or signs that may be HIV-associated

See pages 27–42 for clinical diagnosis and pages 51–53 for communication strategies in this context.

For clinical diagnosis see box on page 31

The patient may be in a group offered screening tests for HIV

Screening will sometimes be offered in a specialist setting, and sometimes in primary care. For example:

For preventing mother-to-child transmission see page 21

- women in antenatal care, in order to prevent mother-to-child transmission
- those found to have conditions which may be associated with HIV (such as TB, lymphoma, hepatitis B or C, syphilis or other STIs) – but

bear in mind that specialist clinics sometimes omit the offer of an HIV test to patients with HIV-associated conditions.

It is important that the value of the HIV test is explained to the patient.

See NICE (2011) *HIV testing: increasing uptake in black Africans* [PH33] and *HIV testing: increasing uptake in men who have sex with men* [PH 34] These will be superceded in December 2016 by new NICE guidelines on HIV testing.

Areas in the UK with high local diagnosed HIV prevalence (greater than two in 1,000 15–59 year olds)

Whilst screening for HIV in higher prevalence areas has been evaluated for newly registering patients in general practice, at the time of writing cost-benefit evaluation has not been published. Such a programme has therefore not yet been systematically commissioned and implemented across the UK. In the meantime, some practices in high prevalence areas offer HIV screening to all newly registering patients and all practitioners in such areas should have a low threshold for offering HIV tests. NICE recommends that where more than 2 in 1000 population have been diagnosed with HIV, all health practitioners should offer and recommend an HIV test to anyone who has a blood test (regardless of the reason). Patients admitted for acute medical care are increasingly likely to be offered an HIV test as routine.

Opportunities to raise the subject of an HIV test may arise:

- before a sexual history has been taken – perhaps in a contraception or cervical screening consultation
- once a sexual history has been taken – perhaps the patient has identified risk factors for HIV
- when a history of injecting drug use has been identified
- in a new patient check during a discussion about sexual health
- if your practice is in an area of high local HIV prevalence.

Remember to emphasise the benefits of earlier HIV diagnosis.

Useful phrases to help bring up HIV testing

If the patient has signs and symptoms of infection ▶

Illnesses like this are usually caused by viruses, for example the glandular fever or flu virus. Some quite rare viruses can also be a cause, and it is important that I don't miss them if they occur. I don't know if you are at risk, but HIV is one of these.

The problems that you have had recently are quite common, and usually minor. However, very occasionally they can give a clue that your immune system is not working as well as it should.

I don't know if you are at risk of HIV, but this is one condition that can affect the immune system. Could I ask you some questions to see if you could be at risk?

From what you tell me you are quite unlikely to have HIV but I think it would be wise to do a test anyway so that we can be sure. Is that OK?

If the patient is in a group offered screening, or a group at higher risk of HIV infection ▶

All pregnant women are automatically offered a test for syphilis, hepatitis B, HIV and rubella – however we think it's better to have this information before you get pregnant. Would you like a test?

Current advice is that everyone who has injected drugs in the past should be offered a test for HIV, because this condition responds so well to treatment. Have you ever considered having a test?

[To a patient with an STI, eg herpes or warts] I would always recommend chlamydia and HIV tests, as you may have been at risk of these infections too – and they are treatable.

If the patient is in a group offered screening, or a group at higher risk of HIV infection (cont'd) ▶

[To a male patient] Because two of your partners in the last year have been male, it is possible that you are at higher risk of HIV. Have you ever considered having an HIV test?

We find that quite a lot of young men are at risk of having sexual health problems. Could I ask you a few questions to see if you are at risk?

OK, so you'd like a test for chlamydia. Would you like an HIV test too?

So you had a negative test for HIV a year ago – is there any reason you wouldn't want another check now?

There is a lot of HIV in your home country, I think. Do you know anyone who is affected? Have you ever had a test?

As part of general holistic care and 'good doctoring' ▶

We are trying to do a lot more HIV testing because undiagnosed HIV can do a lot of damage and we know the infection responds so well to treatment.

There is really quite a lot of undiagnosed HIV in this area so we are trying to increase our testing rates as people do much better if they know they have it.

We include an HIV test in our new patient check for everyone because we're in a part of the country where there are higher than average levels of HIV and we wouldn't want to miss anyone. Is that OK?

As part of general holistic care (cont'd) ▼

> **But doctor – do you really think I need to have an HIV test?**

> **Well I don't wish to dissuade anyone from having an HIV test at present. Currently doctors are doing too few tests, not too many. I would say: if in doubt, test.**

3. The pre-test discussion

The primary purpose of the pre-test discussion is to establish informed consent to the HIV test. Lengthy pre-test counselling is not required unless a patient requests or needs it. The time a discussion takes is extremely variable, but in a well-informed, reasonably low risk person it is likely to take just a minute or less.

Essential elements of the pre-test discussion
The benefits of HIV testing

If the patient gets a negative HIV test result:
- they have the reassurance that they do not have HIV
- they can continue to take steps to avoid HIV.

If the patient gets a positive HIV test result:
- there are very effective treatments that will keep them well and reduce the risk of onward transmission to others
- they can take additional steps to avoid passing on HIV, such as use of condoms or avoiding sharing of needles
- treatment for any other conditions may need to be adjusted
- women can be prevented from passing HIV to their children if they know their status early
- they will have more control over who to tell, and when, than if they find out while very ill.

IMPORTANT!

The essential aspects that need to be covered in the pre-test discussion are:
- the benefits of testing for the individual
- details of how the result will be given.

Check whether you have their contact details

Check the contact details are correct, and ask their preferred method of contact and any possible problems with leaving messages or talking. You will be glad of this if the patient fails to attend for a result that turned out to be positive.

Confirm how results are to be obtained

See BASHH/ MEDFASH (2014) *Standards for the management of sexually transmitted infections (STIs)*

As HIV testing in primary care has hugely increased, it has become normalised. Most practices will use the usual practice system for informing patients of negative results. Then, if an HIV test proves positive, an alternative plan can be made (for example the patient can be contacted and given an urgent appointment with their doctor).

A 'no news is good news' policy is not considered good practice for HIV and STI test results, according to the British Association for Sexual Health and HIV.

Check whether the patient has given clear consent to HIV (or other) tests

Informed consent must be obtained before any test. Ask them directly if they agree to the HIV test. Written consent is not required.

Other areas sometimes covered in a pre-test discussion

See HIV testing aide-memoire on page 96

Given here is a breakdown of further issues that might be covered in a pre-test discussion with a patient who needs or requests it. Not all areas will need to be covered with all patients. A checklist is given on page 96 which can be used as an aide-memoire by the GP or practice nurse.

i) Check the patient's understanding of HIV

Assess their understanding of different transmission routes and of the difference between HIV and AIDS. Some patients believe that if they have had any blood tests in the past, they will automatically have been tested for HIV. Also, the patient should understand the significance of the window period and that a repeat test may be needed.

ii) Discuss risk to date

Knowing the nature of the risk enables you to tailor advice on risk reduction, and knowing the timing of risk(s) is important when considering the window period of the test to be used (see pages 15–17). If doubt about the window period arrange a repeat test at the appropriate interval.

If the patient does not wish to discuss their risk, but wishes to go ahead with a test, they should be able to do so as long as the benefits of discussing risk have been mentioned.

iii) Discuss future risk and risk reduction

This may be the first opportunity that a patient has had to discuss risk reduction. It is best to discuss safer sexual practices and safer injecting practices before the test i) because risks may be taken before the patient is next seen and ii) because a patient is unlikely to be seen simply to be given a negative result so your opportunity to discuss risk is when the test is arranged. If a repeat test is to be arranged, emphasise that if HIV is transmitted between now and the next test, it may not show up in that result. Also, if the patient has recently been exposed, and therefore possibly recently infected, they may well be highly infectious so they should be encouraged to consider this and practise risk reduction before the repeat test.

See more on the timing of risks on page 16

iv) Address the concerns of more vulnerable patients

Ask the patient to consider who knows they are having a test, and who it is safe to tell. Advise the patient not to drink alcohol or take recreational drugs on the day of the result. Consider whether there is any written information that should be given to the patient.

Exploring the implications of a positive test is an important component of pre-test discussions with more vulnerable patients. How are they likely to react if the result is positive? What would their main concerns be if they tested positive? Who would they tell? Who would they not tell? What will be the reactions of those they might tell? What might be the implications for their partner? For their work?

In people with psychological or emotional problems, or those with additional counselling needs, a referral to GUM services for testing may be appropriate. This should be balanced against the benefits of having a test conducted in familiar surroundings and by a clinician known to the patient.

Bear in mind that a small minority of patients may tell you that a positive HIV test result would be too much to bear and they might self-harm in some way. It is important to use your judgement about whether a test in general practice under these circumstances is appropriate, or if the patient may benefit from the additional support that a test in GUM could offer.

v) Explain confidentiality

Explain that a positive test result will need to be recorded in their medical records so that their healthcare remains safe and appropriate. Reassure the patient that such records are stored securely and are only available to the relevant healthcare professionals.

If the patient has concerns about how HIV testing might affect insurance applications:

- explain that a positive result would have to be disclosed to insurance companies if requested
- emphasise that negative tests should not affect insurance applications.

vi) Consider whether other tests are appropriate

It may be appropriate to request other tests at the same time as HIV. For example:

- Patients from countries with a high prevalence of HIV will often also benefit from other tests such as viral hepatitis screening; and, in women of childbearing age or children, haemoglobinopathy testing or checks for rubella immunity may be needed
- if the risk is considered to be due to needle sharing, talk to the patient about testing for hepatitis B and C
- if the risk is unprotected sexual intercourse – particularly if the risk appears high – then you may wish to discuss tests for other STIs such as chlamydia or hepatitis B.

There is a growing trend for routine screening for hepatitis B and C for those from higher prevalence areas. Consider the need for immunisation against hepatitis B.

vii) Consider whether repeat tests will be required

For more detail on the window period see pages 15–17

Ensure the patient understands if they are going to need a repeat test (to cover the window period) before HIV infection can be ruled out.

viii) Check if the patient has a supply of appropriate condoms and lubricant

Some practices can provide condoms and lubricant, but if not, signposting to GUM, contraceptive services or gay men's health organisations where free condoms and lubricant are available is helpful.

4. Giving the result

- **If the result is negative**, you need to consider whether the patient needs a further test because of the window period.
- **If the result is positive**, there are many things you need to consider before the patient attends.

Preparing to give a positive result

You will have time to collect your thoughts and seek advice, because the lab is likely to phone the result through and ask for a repeat sample.

IMPORTANT!
When giving a negative result, don't forget to reinforce advice about minimising risk, if appropriate.

Remember:

- you already have skills in discussing very difficult things
- the patient chose you to do their test, so they chose you to give them the result.

Review the notes from the consultation when you took the test. If the pre-test discussion was brief, there may not be very much information, so prepare to ask the patient to consider the following:
- what is their main concern should the test be positive?
- who knows they were being tested?
- where do they get support?
- is there a partner whose needs you should discuss with the patient? (Formal partner notification should be addressed by the HIV clinic.)

Consider referral arrangements:

See 'the newly diagnosed patient' on page 62

- the patient will need to be referred to a specialist HIV clinic for assessment within two weeks of testing positive so an appointment can be made in advance. Patients may have their own preferences for treatment centres so should be involved in this decision wherever possible
- have phone numbers of support organisations and relevant literature available.

When the patient attends

Give the result soon after the patient is in the room and has sat down. Delaying disclosure can heighten anxiety. This allows you more time to attend to and deal with the patient's reactions. Some patients are expecting a positive result and may be quite calm. Indeed, some may have already come to terms with being positive. A calm exterior can also mask a sense of shock.

In the case of a positive result, listen carefully and make the discussion focused and tailored to the individual.

You should emphasise the positive aspects: patients are better off knowing that they have HIV.

When the consultation is coming to an end:
- give the patient the details of any appointment that you have arranged
- remember that risk reduction advice to protect partners will need to be addressed at some point, but this may be hard for the patient to take in at this consultation
- arrange to follow up the patient within a few days as they may well have additional questions and it will give you the opportunity to check that referral to the specialist service has been actioned

case study

An opportunity to test for HIV

Pascal, aged 26, attended the practice nurse for a new patient check. He was an accountant, and generally fit and well with no significant past medical history. The practice encouraged sexual health promotion, and the nurse raised the subject after other aspects of the check were complete.

She asked him if it was okay if she asked questions to see if he could be at risk of any sexual health problems. He agreed, but seemed to become a bit guarded. The nurse took a partner history according to her routine, avoiding assumptions. The patient opened up and relaxed, and shortly explained that he wasn't living alone as he had told her, but was gay and living with his partner of three years. He felt this relationship was mutually monogamous, but he had had several partners prior to this. She asked about condom use and established that he had had significant risk of exposure to HIV through several 'casual' sexual contacts in years gone by. Pascal explained that he had always meant to have a test for HIV, but never got round to it. He had also discussed it with his partner in the past, but more recently the subject had been forgotten.

After discussion it was agreed that Pascal would suggest to his partner that he also registered 'as it seems a really nice practice'. The nurse agreed she would be happy to arrange an HIV test for both of them. In due course, both attended. The HIV tests were negative. They were very grateful to the nurse for having dealt with an issue that had been a suppressed but niggling worry.

> The HIV tests were negative. They were very grateful to the nurse for having dealt with an issue that had been a suppressed but niggling worry.

Learning points:
- Offering the HIV test can allay anxiety even where the result is negative.
- A negative result is a good opportunity for sexual health promotion.

Summary: how to improve HIV detection in your practice

Familiarise GPs and practice nurses in the team with:

- the more HIV-specific aspects of primary HIV infection, and be ready to ask about them in patients with a 'glandular fever-like' illness (pages 28–29)
- those urgent conditions that may present in patients whose HIV infection remains undiagnosed, most importantly PCP (pages 31–32)
- those indicator conditions that are associated with HIV infection (pages 31–40), especially if they have had:
  - more than one in the last two to three years; or
  - an unusually difficult to treat or severe form of these conditions
- risk factors for HIV which should prompt an offer of an HIV test (see pages 48–49).

Print off the clinical indicator conditions table in the reference section at the back of this booklet (page 105) and put it up in all consulting rooms.

Plan and practise strategies for discussing HIV with patients in different clinical circumstances.

Take steps to incorporate HIV testing into the health promotion work of the practice nurse team.

Consider including the HIV test in all new patient registrations if local diagnosed HIV prevalence is equal to or greater than two in 1,000.

Arrange a practice development session on HIV and STI testing – your local GUM service could help, or look at online learning options such as:

- e-GP, through the RCGP
- HIVTIPs – an educational web tool from MEDFASH for GPs and practice nurses, with individual and group exercises, to help them and their teams increase HIV testing

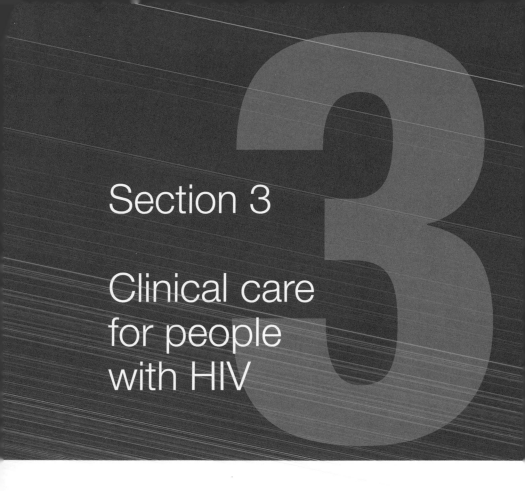

Section 3

Clinical care for people with HIV

IN THIS SECTION

Clinical care for people with HIV

HIV is increasingly managed as a chronic disease, with most people living a near-normal life span. Care will involve a partnership between the patient, primary care and specialist centres.

Patients with HIV

1 The newly diagnosed patient

Unfortunately, HIV infection is still a stigmatising condition and thus telling friends, family or colleagues is never easy. Some people will not be prepared to absorb fully the news of a positive test result. Some may need considerable support over time.

A significant number of women with HIV have been identified through antenatal screening. These women may face a truly challenging range of issues: a newly diagnosed and serious medical condition; starting life-long medication; a pregnancy; and the possibility that existing children and/or their partner are infected – all at the same time.

2. The patient who informs you they have HIV

A patient may inform their GP or practice nurse that they have HIV. Many patients with long-standing HIV infection can be considered 'expert patients' and some of these may be proactive in involving you in their general medical care.

Others may be more anxious about divulging this information. It may take some time before a patient with HIV chooses to disclose this to their GP, or they may find that illness forces the decision. They may require reassurance about the confidentiality of their records and the attitudes of practice staff who will need to know about their HIV status. Communication with the specialist clinic should be established as soon as possible.

Health promotion, screening and immunisation for people with HIV

1. HIV metabolic abnormalities and cardiovascular risk

People living with HIV are at higher risk of metabolic abnormalities including dyslipidaemia and insulin resistance. The mechanisms and role of therapy versus other risk factors are still debated. Of particular importance is cardiovascular disease – as such, a lower threshold of suspicion and investigation of cardiovascular disease is warranted in those with HIV. Effort should be put into promoting healthy diets, exercise, alcohol control, blood pressure checks and smoking cessation. There are no recorded interactions between ART and varenicline. If in doubt seek expert advice and check on line: www.hiv-druginteractions.org.

2. Cervical screening

See case study
page 65

Women with HIV are more at risk from HPV-related disease, including cervical cancer and warts. Currently women with HIV infection should have annual smears, and will be recommended to have more frequent follow-up and colposcopy if abnormalities are found. Women on ART, with normal immunity and without high risk HPV infection, may have a normal level of risk, although guidance for this group has not yet changed.

3. Immunisation

See Public Health
England
*Immunisation
against infectious
disease*

The practice can and should play a key role in immunising patients who have HIV. Current advice can be found in the *BHIVA Guidelines on the use of vaccines in HIV-positive adults* (2015) which are very useful and practical for GPs, or the summary of their recommendations endorsed by the RCGP, also available on the BHIVA website. 'The Green Book' (Public Health England: *Immunisation against infectious disease*) has up to date advice on immunisation, including a section on immunosuppression in Chapter 6, and a list of contraindications to each immunisation used. This can be viewed online.

See *BHIVA Guidelines
on the use of
vaccines in HIV-
positive adults 2015*

Individuals with HIV infection should not normally receive BCG, cholera, or oral typhoid. Live oral polio (Sabin) immunisation should not be given to patients or their children (if a parent or carer is immunosuppressed) due to the small risk of contact with excreted live vaccine. All inactivated immunisations such as pertussis, diphtheria, tetanus, *inactivated* polio (Salk), typhoid, and meningitis C are safe. This is an example where regular communication between the GP and the specialist team can pay dividends.

Adults with HIV should be offered:
- influenza immunisation each year
- hepatitis B testing and immunisation as appropriate (it is important to

check hepatitis B titres post-immunisation and seek specialist advice for those who do not respond, see BHIVA Guidelines, above).

- hepatitis A immunisation for men who have sex with men
- pneumococcal vaccination – please see latest *BHIVA guidelines on the use of vaccines in HIV positive adults* as to differing indications and administration regimens for the use of PCV or PPV vaccinations.

In addition, those aged over 60 years, and with a CD4 count above 200, should be offered varicella zoster (shingles) immunisation.

Specialist advice should be sought from the paediatric team about immunisation of children infected with HIV, and children of parents with HIV.

If a baby is born to a mother with HIV, transmitted infection will usually have been identified by eight weeks. Inactivated polio should be given if any family members are immunosuppressed, or if there is doubt about the baby's status.

> Check for drug interactions at:
> www.hiv-druginteractions.org

4. Advice for international travel

Check the entry requirements for the country concerned to ensure they do not deny entry to those with HIV (check www.hivtravel.org).

Hepatitis A and B vaccination should be offered as appropriate (see 3. Immunisation above). Check the most up-to-date *BHIVA guidelines on the use of vaccines in HIV-positive adults* for recommendations regarding yellow fever vaccine.

Malaria prophylaxis is used, but interactions with ART can occur. The agents, ritonavir and cobicistat, for example, can interact with several antimalarials. Check on the invaluable (and easy to use) www.hiv-druginteractions.org website for drug interaction information. Larger HIV clinics have specialist pharmacists, who can give advice.

Advice on safer sex and the avoidance of sexually transmitted infections may need to be reinforced for travellers.

Patients may also be offered a concise medical summary, including prescribed medication, in case of illness abroad. Some drugs (eg opiates) may need a licence from the Home Office.

> **USEFUL INFO**
>
> Some countries restrict entry for those with HIV. Patients should check with the relevant embassy or embassies before planning their trip. See www.hivtravel.org for a list of these countries.

case study

A case of missing smears?

Consuela is a 40-year-old woman from South America who registered with the practice in 2004. She had moved to the UK some 13 years previously and had been under the care of another practice in the locality, but switched when she changed address. Consuela was already aware of her positive HIV status when she registered, but did not disclose this to the practice. Over the next two years she did not attend the surgery very often and did not respond to invitations for cervical screening. The practice nurse had tried frequently to call her in. On the phone on one occasion Consuela told the practice nurse that a smear test had been done in a 'clinic appointment' at the hospital. The nurse asked her to bring a copy of the result but this was not forthcoming.

In 2007 Consuela became pregnant and was duly referred to the antenatal unit at the same hospital where she was accessing her HIV care. The pregnancy was uncomplicated and she delivered a girl by normal delivery. The baby has also since been registered with the practice and she has been fully vaccinated; she is HIV-negative.

In 2009 an unexpected hospital smear result arrived at the practice showing severe squamous dyskaryosis present with features suspicious of invasion; colposcopy was recommended. There had been no symptoms. Within six weeks a radical hysterectomy had been performed with lymph node dissection, although there was evidence of micro-invasion confirmed on histology. Consuela is under the close supervision of the gynaecologist and the specialist oncology unit. This year Consuela has had her first post-operative vaginal vault smear which shows moderate squamous dyskaryosis and it is likely that she will need chemotherapy. This is being planned.

Learning points
- Women with HIV are at higher risk of cervical cancer and should have annual screening tests.
- Practices should liaise closely with HIV clinics to ensure the tests have been done and results are available.

Sexual and reproductive health

1. Sexual health advice

For more, see
BASHH/BHIVA/FSRH
(2008) *UK
guidelines for the
management of
sexual and
reproductive health
of people living with
HIV infection*

Healthcare workers need to be able to discuss sex and sexual practices with patients living with HIV. Many people find it difficult to maintain safer sex, so practitioners should be supportive and avoid criticism. Ideally, practices should provide condoms and (for anal sex) lubricant, but if not, signposting to services which provide free supplies is helpful.

Support from an expert counsellor or health adviser can help address difficulties related to HIV disclosure, or assist with adopting or maintaining safer sexual behaviour. Expert advice may also be needed to address concerns about the (albeit unlikely) possibility of criminal prosecution if HIV transmission occurs.

For evidence of
effectiveness of ART
as prevention, see
BHIVA and the
Expert Advisory
Group on AIDS
(EAGA) *Position
statement on the
use of antiretroviral
therapy to reduce
HIV transmission.*
September 2014

Transmission of HIV is dramatically reduced when a patient takes their ART regularly and once the viral load is suppressed. Knowledge of this can reduce anxiety. Nevertheless use of condoms (which also prevent other STIs) is still recommended.

The most recent national guidance no longer recommends post-exposure prophylaxis following sexual exposure (PEPSE) in the event of unprotected sexual intercourse with an HIV positive person who has a sustained undetectable viral load. However it may have a role in the partners of patients with adherence problems, or whose viral loads are unsuppressed or being actively monitored (for a number of possible reasons). See page 87 for more information.

For detailed advice
on safer sex, see
BASHH/BHIVA
(2012) *UK national
guidelines on safer
sex advice*

The presence of STIs in either partner may increase the risk of HIV transmission, further compounding the importance of continued condom use, and it is important to offer STI screening regularly to people living with HIV and their partners. This is especially important if either partner is non-monogamous.

Hepatitis C has become epidemic among a subgroup of men with HIV who have sex with men, between whom it is mostly sexually transmitted and often associated with 'chemsex' (the use of certain stimulant and disinhibiting drugs to facilitate and enhance sex). It is therefore also important to check for other blood-borne viruses. Superinfection with a drug-resistant strain of HIV (thus limiting future treatment options) is also possible, although this has been observed far less frequently than initially anticipated.

2. Contraception

As for all women, the most effective methods of contraception should always be recommended as first line to minimise risk of unplanned pregnancy. Contraceptive choice for HIV-infected women may be limited by interactions with ART although this is becoming less of a concern as there is a move away from the use of protease inhibitors and NNRTIs

See Faculty of Sexual and Reproductive Healthcare (updated 2012) *Clinical Guidance: Drug Interactions with Hormonal Contraception*

towards integrase inhibitors which have far fewer interactions. (See page 73 for details of antiretroviral drugs.) Condoms are a useful additional precaution against pregnancy where the efficacy of the primary contraceptive choice may be reduced.

Clinical decisions about individual patients can be greatly supported by use of the www.hiv-druginteractions.org website, although at times the site simply confirms the lack of evidence in this field. Below we summarise some of the main points.

Contraceptives affected by enzyme inducing drugs

Combined oral contraception (COC), the combined transdermal patch, combined vaginal ring, progestogen-only pill (POP) and progestogen-only implant may have reduced efficacy with some antiretroviral combinations (including some first-line combinations) due to enzyme induction, and expert advice should be sought. Condoms are advised as failure has been reported. Newer drugs such as the integrase inhibitors raltegravir, dolutegravir and elvitegravir do not interact with steroid hormones but may be used in combination with other ART which does. There is little published data on the pharmacokinetics of oestrogen and progestogens used with patients on ART. A cautious approach is wise.

Contraceptives not affected by enzyme inducing drugs

The efficacy of the IUD (intrauterine device), the IUS (intrauterine system) or depot medroxyprogesterone acetate injections (at the usual intervals) does not appear to be affected by enzyme inducing drugs and these should always be offered as first choice to women taking enzyme inducing drugs.

Emergency contraception

See Faculty of Sexual and Reproductive Healthcare (2016) *UK Medical Eligibility Criteria for Contraceptive Use*

The copper IUD is the most effective method and also efficacy will not be affected by drug interactions.

Doubling the dose of levonorgestrel (*Levonelle*) is generally advised for women on medication that interacts with progestogens (efavirenz, nevirapine, most protease inhibitors) although this is unlicensed. For women on other antiretrovirals this is not necessary; if in doubt a double dose may be appropriate as levonorgestrel side effects are few.

In the absence of any data on its use by women taking enzyme inducing drugs, doubling the dose of ulipristal acetate (*ellaOne*) is currently not advised. Ulipristal acetate should not be used by women using enzyme inducing drugs or who have stopped them within the last four weeks.

The *UK Medical Eligibility Criteria for Contraceptive Use* provide detailed guidance on other personal or medical factors which aids safe contraceptive prescribing. Further information and up-to-date advice should always be sought from specialist services if there is uncertainty.

3. Fertility and assisted conception

Some couples in which one partner has HIV will want to start a family. This is an area which will be managed by specialists, but it is useful to have some knowledge of the options to discuss with patients, should they raise the matter.

For fertility advice when individuals are HIV positive, see National Institute for Health and Care Excellence (NICE) guideline CG156 (2013) *Fertility problems: assessment and treatment*

Options for couples hoping to conceive include:
i)   Careful adherence to ART, with confirmed viral suppression and acceptance of a very small risk of transmission
ii) Timing of unprotected sex to ovulation only, to reduce the frequency of exposure (and thus the risk)
iii) Ensuring the absence of other STIs
iv) Consideration of prophylaxis therapy for the non-HIV infected partner (unnecessary in the context of a suppressed viral load in the HIV-positive partner).

In these circumstances the risk of transmission is very low, although the risk of virus being present in the semen cannot be entirely ruled out.

Other options where the male partner is HIV-positive include:
v) Sperm washing. This was once considered the gold standard for couples where the man is HIV-positive and the woman negative. However, it is no longer recommended if the man is on HIV treatment with an undetectable viral load. Eligibility for NHS funding for this is decided locally.
vi) Donor insemination.

Where the female partner is HIV-positive:
vii) Self insemination with her partner's semen. Fertility clinics can provide equipment/quills. Ovulation kits may be used in addition to optimise the timing of insemination.

All couples planning pregnancy should discuss their options with their HIV physician.

Investigation and treatment of sub-fertility in people living with HIV should be as for the uninfected population.

4. Antenatal and postnatal care

Many women with HIV are well and actively choose pregnancy. Some may have an unplanned pregnancy that they choose to continue. Some may have undergone the traumatic experience of discovering through antenatal HIV testing that they are infected with HIV.

Managing the pregnancy of a woman with HIV is strongly influenced by the need to prevent transmission to the baby. The risk of transmission can be reduced from around 20 per cent to well under 1 per cent by use of:

- ART in pregnancy, covering delivery
- a short course of ART for the baby
- vaginal delivery for women on ART with an undetectable viral load; elective caesarean section for others
- avoidance of breastfeeding.

Support of bottle feeding

See BHIVA (2014) Guidelines for the management of HIV infection in pregnant women 2012 (2014 interim review)

Although there is evidence that ART reduces HIV viral load in breast milk, the complete avoidance of breastfeeding for infants born to mothers with HIV is still recommended in the UK, regardless of maternal disease status and viral load. (This is not the advice in resource poor settings where the risk of harm from formula feeding is greater). Support for bottle feeding should be offered and GPs may be able to prescribe infant formula milk if they feel it is appropriate. This advice is not accepted by all mothers with HIV, not least because the avoidance of breastfeeding may provoke enquiries about the reasons, leading to unwanted speculation about (or even disclosure of) the mother's HIV status. Where such concerns arise, advice and support should be available from midwives and others involved in care.

In the rare instances where a mother with HIV who is on effective ART with a repeatedly undetectable viral load chooses to breastfeed, intensive support and monitoring of mother and baby are recommended.

Asylum seekers

Asylum seekers identified as HIV-positive (commonly through antenatal screening) face particular financial difficulties. Asylum support regulations allow a payment of an extra £3 a week to be made for children up to three years (£5 for under-ones) who are being supported by the UK Border Agency to help with the purchase of healthy foods. Pregnant women who are being supported by the UK Border Agency can also receive £3 a week under this scheme for the duration of their pregnancy.

Mental health

See British Psychological Society, BHIVA & MEDFASH (2011) Standards for psychological support for adults living with HIV

Mental health problems are more common in people with HIV than in the general population. There are several possible explanations. Firstly, those with pre-existing mental health problems are often more vulnerable and may have been prone to engaging in high-risk sex or injecting drugs in the past. Secondly, those diagnosed with HIV can face stigma, isolation and discrimination, all of which may make them more likely to become depressed or anxious. Many chronic conditions are in any case associated with an increased risk of depression. Finally, some HIV drugs

case study

A long-term survivor

Andy is a 53-year-old gay man who has been living with HIV since 1989. He has a previous diagnosis of PCP and CMV retinitis and is visually impaired from this. He had a successful career, but when he became unwell with AIDS he gave up his job and has not worked since. He has a long antiretroviral history and has suffered from many side-effects over the years including renal stones and renal impairment from indinavir, marked lipoatrophy and lipodystrophy, which he found very stigmatising, and problematic GI side-effects which he has to manage symptomatically. He is currently stable on a complex ART regimen with an undetectable viral load and a CD4 count of 367/µl. He has multiple drug resistance because of his long antiretroviral history and has limited antiretroviral options at present. He is also on medication for raised cholesterol and hypertension, and he has impaired glucose tolerance. He is therefore taking an increasing list of non-HIV medication as well.

He suffered multiple bereavements in the 1980s losing many friends and his partner to AIDS. His family are aware of his HIV diagnosis, but live a long way from him; he has few friends and is very isolated due to his chronic ill health and inability to work. He has had several significant episodes of depression since being diagnosed with HIV. He feels quite bleak and negative about his future and his depression responds in part to SSRIs (selective serotonin reuptake inhibitors).

He has made attempts to get back into employment, but is hampered by his poor vision and lack of work throughout the1990s. He presents a challenge on many levels to his GP, with whom he has a good relationship and whom he sees frequently.

> He presents a challenge on many levels to his GP, with whom he has a good relationship and whom he sees frequently.

Learning points

- The mental health problems experienced by people with HIV are similar to those seen in people coping with a range of chronic conditions or disabilities.
- Management of mental health problems is as normal in general practice, with the proviso that prescribed medications need to be checked for interactions with ART.

can be associated with mental health symptoms.

Some HIV services in larger urban areas have access to psychiatrists and psychologists who specialise in this area. For the GP, management of mental health problems should be as normal.

Managing HIV-related problems

1. The GP's role

For more, see BHIVA (2013) *Standards of care for people living with HIV 2013*

In many ways, looking after someone with HIV is no different from looking after those with other chronic conditions. The specialist centres are responsible for initiating and monitoring ART and they remain responsible for prescribing it. The role of the GP will vary depending upon the health of the patient. In addition, the relationship the GP has with the patient, and the relationship between the patient and their specialist team, will affect how primary care is used. For many health problems, all that is needed is advice, reassurance or simple treatment. Nevertheless, there are times when immediate referral for assessment is likely to be appropriate.

It is important for GPs to have effective communication with the HIV specialists looking after the patient and their family. HIV clinics should inform GPs about current HIV medication, problems and test results, and in return GPs should be prepared to notify specialists if there are significant changes in the patient's management, medication or circumstances. It is also good practice to copy the HIV specialist into letters to/from other specialties as appropriate. Internal referrals from the HIV specialists should also be copied to the GP so that all clinicians involved are kept informed.

ART has had an enormous impact on morbidity and mortality from HIV disease. Your patient (particularly if recently infected) has a good chance of achieving normal or near normal life expectancy so long as he/she is adherent to the medication and clinically responding. Here we give an overview of clinical management. In the next section we explain how the drugs act.

2. A general approach to new presentations of health problems

Physical problems caused by HIV infection are significantly less common in the diagnosed patient now that ART is widely used. A patient with HIV who presents with symptoms might have:

See side effects of ART pages 76–80

- problems which relate to HIV disease (check the most recent CD4 count)
- side effects or drug interactions due to ART
- an unconnected problem.

You may be able to take the first steps to distinguish which of these is the case. A recent CD4 count that is comfortably above 300 cells/µl, in a patient with a suppressed viral load, makes HIV-related problems less likely. Check which antiretrovirals the patient is on, and check for side effects in the British National Formulary (BNF) and also on page 99. Review whether the patient could have a problem with drug interactions by using the HIV drug interactions website (see page 75) which also notifies about food stuffs and recreational drugs that can interact.

3. Metabolic abnormalities and co-morbidities

People living with HIV are at higher risk of metabolic abnormalities including dyslipidaemia and insulin resistance. There is increased risk of cardiovascular disease – and, as such, a lower threshold of suspicion and investigation of cardiovascular disease is warranted in those with HIV. It is also clear that HIV-positive individuals are at a higher risk of several age-related morbidities including chronic kidney disease and low bone mineral density. As the latter may be due to ART, as well as factors such as lifestyle risks and previous steroid treatment, specialist advice should be sought. Co-morbidities are therefore common in HIV patients and GPs are ideally placed to orchestrate aspects of care.

4. Commoner conditions

For commoner conditions at a glance see pages 100–104

Many more minor HIV-related problems are also common in patients who do not have HIV, for example shingles and seborrhoeic dermatitis. Management of such conditions is generally the same and the GP is likely to be familiar with treatments. However, the immunosuppressed patient may require longer treatment than other patients.

5. Conditions that require urgent referral

For serious conditions associated with HIV see pages 31–37

Serious conditions due to HIV disease affect patients with CD4 counts below 200 cells/µl (except TB, see page 33).

Symptoms that require careful assessment include:
- respiratory
- visual (even if apparently minor, such as floaters)
- progressive or acute neurological problems.

For more, see BHIVA (2015) *BHIVA guidelines for the treatment of HIV-1-positive adults with antiretroviral therapy 2015*

Side effects of ART are sometimes serious or even life-threatening – check which medication the patient is on and liaise with the specialist if you think the patient is developing a serious adverse reaction.

6. Hepatitis B or C co-infection

Viral hepatitis is commoner in those at risk of HIV. Chronic carriage of hepatitis B is more frequent. Re-infection with hepatitis C remains an important area for prevention amongst a sub-group of MSM who have high risk sexual behaviours (including chemsex, see page 91).

For more, see BHIVA (2014) *Management of hepatitis viruses in adults infected with HIV 2013* (updated September 2014)

The management of co-infected patients is complex and rapidly advancing, with control of hepatitis B, and eradication of hepatitis C, as goals. The primary care team can assist with adherence to treatment or offer other support.

Further information can be found on the BHIVA website.

Caring for people on antiretroviral therapy (ART)

1. How the drugs act

Entry inhibitors (EIs)
EIs either block the binding of HIV to cell surface receptors (CCR5 antagonists) or prevent the viral membrane of HIV fusing with the target cell membrane and entering the cell (fusion inhibitors). The use of this drug class is relatively uncommon.

Nucleoside and nucleotide reverse transcriptase inhibitors (NRTIs)
NRTIs inhibit the enzyme reverse transcriptase that is key to transcribing the viral RNA into proviral DNA.

Non-nucleoside reverse transcriptase inhibitors (NNRTIs)
NNRTIs also inhibit the enzyme reverse transcriptase.

Integrase inhibitors (IIs)
IIs block the action of integrase, a viral enzyme that inserts the viral genome into the DNA of the host cell.

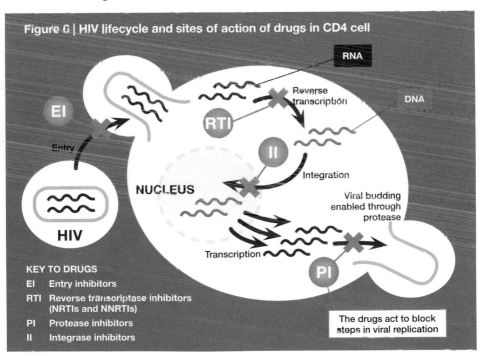

Figure 6 | HIV lifecycle and sites of action of drugs in CD4 cell

Protease inhibitors (PIs)

PIs inhibit the production of protease. Viral protease is needed to form new mature virus particles.

2. Drug combinations used in ART

For a list of drugs see page 97

HIV readily mutates in the process of replication. This means that resistance to most single anti-HIV drugs develops very rapidly. For this reason drugs are usually used in combinations of three or more.

The choice of regimen will depend upon efficacy in viral suppression; the need to minimise side effects and long-term toxicity; patient convenience – and preparations available in the NHS. For some drugs, blood levels are enhanced by using pharmacoenhancers that inhibit the cytochrome P450 metabolism of other components of the combination. This is called 'boosting'. There are two boosters: ritonavir (an old HIV drug given at subtherapeutic doses) and cobicistat. Both are an important cause of drug-drug interactions.

3. When to start ART

For more, see BHIVA (2015) *BHIVA guidelines for the treatment of HIV-1-positive adults with antiretroviral therapy 2015*

Published evidence has supported increasingly early initiation of ART. In recent years initiation had been recommended at a CD4 count of approximately 350 cells/µl, but UK guidelines now simply recommend that people with HIV start ART (without specifying any CD4 count). The clinical priority is to avoid the morbidity associated with late diagnosis and to reduce transmission by lowering infectivity through treatment.

There are a few relatively standard ART starting regimens. Choice will be influenced by a number of factors including co-morbidities, drug-drug interactions and the possibility of viral resistance.

4. Monitoring progress

Monitoring of ART is primarily by viral load (see pages 17–18). The aim is to reduce the viral load to undetectable levels, usually within three to six months of starting therapy. A persistently high viral load will either be due to non-adherence, or to the development of drug resistance.

5. Drug resistance

Resistance of the virus to ART is minimised if combination therapy is maintained at therapeutic levels in the blood stream. Drug resistance can be provoked by, for example, non-adherence to medication or drug-drug interactions and, once established, is irreversible. Cross-resistance between classes of drugs means treatment choices are further limited.

6. Adherence to ART regimens

If people with, say, hypertension miss their medication for a short period of time, it will still be effective when they re-start. Unfortunately this is not always the case with ART due to the development of viral resistance. How many days can be missed depends on the regimen, but the risks of developing resistance increase greatly, even with the most 'forgiving' regimens, after missing two days. Risks from missing a small amount of medication decrease if the patient has already been stably virally suppressed for many months or for years.

IMPORTANT!
Adherence is essential to prevent drug resistance developing.

Therefore adherence to a long-term drug regimen is one of the biggest challenges to those who live with HIV as well as to those who support them. Monitoring, and supporting, adherence is something the primary care team can do well. When the patient is seen, the GP or practice nurse should assess how they are coping with taking their medication and whether they are missing doses. Patients need to understand the reasons behind the requirement for optimal adherence as well as the possible consequences of repeated missed doses. If they do discontinue, or carry on having difficulty with adherence, try to explore the reasons.

Where possible, once-a-day combination preparations are prescribed If such preparations cannot be used, specialists will try to devise other practical regimens. However the timing of the medication through the day may be complex, especially if medications for other conditions are also taken. For example some might need to be taken well in advance of eating, and others directly after.

Even without these practical complications, it is hard to sustain any regular regimen without losing motivation or even simply forgetting doses.

In some areas HIV specialists can arrange adherence support.

7. Drug interactions

PIs and NNRTIs are the groups most affected by drug interactions, being metabolised via the cytochrome P450 enzyme system in the liver. These interactions can lead to both increased toxicity and decreased efficacy. Dietary substances, herbal remedies and recreational drugs can all interact significantly. GPs should be very cautious, as atypical interactions can occur: for example ritonavir can block the metabolism of inhaled or intranasal fluticasone so effectively that the patient can develop iatrogenic Cushing's syndrome. Always check!

Check for drug interactions at:
www.hiv-druginteractions.org

The internationally renowned website www.hiv-druginteractions.org, run by the University of Liverpool, includes information on interactions between antiretrovirals and most other medications, as well as dietary substances (under herbals/supplements/vitamins) and recreational drugs (under illicit/recreational). There is an option to submit individual queries. In some areas advice from specialist pharmacists linked to hospital HIV services is available.

8. ART side effects

There has been a shift away from the antiretrovirals associated with the most serious side effects and so these are now a great deal less frequent, strengthening further the major advantages of ART. Side effects are most common with the three older drug classes, NRTIs, NNRTIs and PIs. Integrase inhibitors are largely well tolerated as is maraviroc, the main entry inhibitor in use. For a full list of both serious and minor side effects, see the BNF. See 'Quick reference' page 97 to identify which group each drug is in and page 99 for a table of side effects by drug type. Don't forget that drug and substance interactions (www.hiv-druginteractions.org) may be an underlying cause of side effects.

> For ART side effects at a glance see page 99

As ART should not be stopped without good reason, management should always be discussed with a specialist before action is taken.

Minor side effects

> Check the *BNF* for side effects

ART can cause a range of minor side effects, which are generally listed in the BNF. The GP will often be able to manage minor side effects in the normal way. However, they should always check for drug interactions (see page 75). Symptomatic treatment is given on pages 100–104 (a guide to managing HIV-related problems).

Serious or unusual side effects

Some of the more serious side effects may not be the type of problem that GPs would normally consider could be due to medication, such as osteoporosis or Fanconi syndrome (a renal tubule disorder). In addition, some serious 'unusual' side effects of ART can present in an insidious way, such as lactic acidosis, leaving the GP at risk of overlooking their significance. These are overwhelmingly associated with older antiretrovirals such as nevirapine or abacavir, the use of which has decreased over time.

> Could the problem be caused by a drug interaction? Check www.hiv-druginteractions.org

Hypersensitivity

Hypersensitivity can occur with all drugs to different degrees. Nevirapine (now rarely used) and abacavir are more often associated with serious reactions:

Abacavir. Up to 8 per cent of those who take abacavir will react, and this can be life-threatening. A human leucocyte antigen (HLA) test is used to identify those who are at higher risk of such a reaction, and exclude them from abacavir use. This greatly reduces, but does not eliminate, hypersensitivity reactions which usually occur within the first six weeks of exposure and so patients will be kept under specialist review. Fever or rash are typical, but a range of non-specific symptoms such as vomiting or myalgia are possible. Seek advice urgently if suspected.

Psychiatric problems

Efavirenz is the drug most associated with this group of side effects. It is still used as part of ART regimens. Nightmares, sleep disturbances, mood changes, behaviour changes and vivid (life-like) dreams are common. More severe presentations, including psychosis and suicidal ideation, have been described. Symptoms are generally at the initiation of therapy and transient, but can persist. Other NNRTIs, and the integrase inhibitors, may also cause psychiatric side effects.

Hyperlipidaemia

This varies with different drugs. Rises in cholesterol or triglycerides are sometimes extreme. Older protease inhibitors are most commonly associated, but with varying impact on lipids: lopinavir/ritonavir combinations are currently thought to be the worst. Efavirenz is also associated with an adverse lipid profile, other drugs less so.

Statins (but avoiding simvastatin with antiretroviral boosters due to interactions) and fibrates (bezafibrate) are often used. A change in antiretroviral regimen may be indicated.

IMPORTANT!
Consider hepatic metabolism and interactions when selecting drugs, especially statins.
Simvastatin may be CONTRAINDICATED with ART!

As is the norm, diet and cardiovascular disease (CVD) risk factors (such as hypertension and smoking) should be addressed. Lipids should be monitored routinely. GPs may be ideally placed to do this, and to prescribe an appropriate statin: clinic letters should make responsibilities clear and relevant blood results should be shared.

Lipodystrophy

Lipodystrophy – abnormal fat distribution, potentially caused by any antiretroviral – is an overarching term for two separate presentations: lipoatrophy and lipohypertrophy. These two forms of lipodystrophy may co-exist and may be associated with insulin resistance and hyperlipidaemia.

Lipoatrophy is a loss of subcutaneous fat causing facial thinning and limb and buttock wasting. It is mainly due to early generation NRTIs and is now much less frequently seen. Many patients living with HIV, exposed to these older drugs, have ongoing problems with fat loss.

Lipohypertrophy typically presents as central (truncal) adiposity with an increase in intra-abdominal fat, buffalo hump and breast enlargement. Initially thought to be attributable to PIs, the evidence for association is weakening. Always consider the possibility of drug interactions as a cause of fat redistribution; these can be so potent that several inhaled, intranasal, ocular or topical steroids (such as fluticasone) in combination with the boosters ritonavir or cobicistat can lead to iatrogenic Cushing's syndrome and adrenal failure.

Fear of lipodystrophy, with its marked effects on facial appearance and body shape, may still lead to some patients avoiding or discontinuing ART, even though current antiretrovirals do not cause it. Patients with lipodystrophy may experience stigma and may have low self-esteem, isolation and depression. Treatment for this syndrome is still largely unsatisfactory. A number of specialist centres offer treatment with polylactic acid, a filling agent for facial wasting.

Diabetes (type II)

For ART drugs by class see page 97

Susceptibility to diabetes – probably through insulin resistance – may be associated with ART and will be compounded by obesity. It can be managed in the usual way, but monitoring and additional medication may induce 'adherence fatigue' in some patients. This can impact on both HIV and diabetes. Again, it is important to pay attention to other CVD risk factors in such patients and drug-drug interactions.

Left to right:

1. Lipoatrophy. One of the biggest fears of patients taking ART, this syndrome may also be associated with metabolic abnormalities such as diabetes and hyperlipidaemia.

2. Lipodystrophy. A syndrome probably caused by ART and characterised by redistribution of body fat.

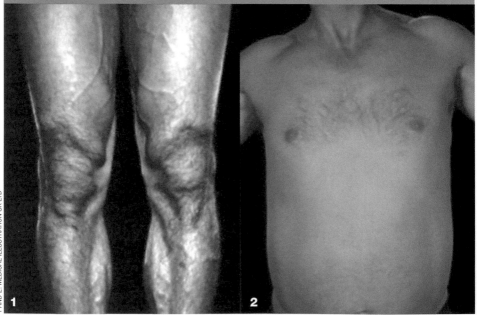

1 AND 2. MEDICAL ILLUSTRATION UK LTD

1

2

Bone density loss

Those with HIV are at higher risk of osteopenia, osteoporosis and fractures. This may be due to a number of factors including lifestyle risks (such as smoking or alcohol), previous steroid treatment and antiretroviral therapy. Many first line ART regimens cause a small decline in bone density; however the drug most closely implicated is the first used formulation of tenofovir (tenofovir disoproxil fumarate, TDF – as opposed to the newer tenofovir alafenamide). If a DEXA (dual energy X-ray absorptiometry) scan confirms density loss and/or the FRAX (Fracture Risk Assessment Tool) score is greater than 20 per cent in any patient with HIV then specialist advice should be sought.

Impact on renal function

The original formulation of tenofovir (tenofovir disoproxil fumarate, TDF) can be associated with an acute or gradual decline in renal function and the patient may need to switch to another drug combination. The newer formulation, tenofovir alafenamide, has a better renal safety profile. Atazanavir is also implicated with renal disease. To complicate matters, several antiretrovirals can cause a rise in serum creatinine via inhibition of tubular transport (ie a rise in creatinine and decline in estimated glomerular filtration rate (GFR) but no change in true GFR). If this is neither progressive nor associated with tubular dysfunction then standard monitoring is appropriate.

Ureteric colic, renal and ureteric stones

Atazanavir is the PI most commonly associated with these side effects, but others are also implicated.

Lactic acidosis

This condition is strongly associated with older NRTIs (which some patients are on, if initiated outside the UK) and rarely occurs with newer members of this group. A potentially life-threatening problem, it may present with non-specific symptoms such as nausea, loss of appetite or abdominal pain. In clear-cut cases patients will be obviously unwell – acidotic and with hepatomegaly. Deranged liver function and raised serum lactate may be found. Such patients need hospital admission and full review of their ART regimen.

Hepatic toxicity

All antiretrovirals have the potential to cause hepatotoxicity, whether as part of lactic acidosis, a hypersensitivity reaction or for other reasons. Broadly speaking IIs seem less associated with hepatotoxicity than NRTIs, NNRTIs and PIs. Patients with hepatitis B or C co-infection are at higher risk.
    Atazanavir commonly causes an unconjugated hyperbilirubinaemia,

case study

The dangers of being unaware of a patient's HIV treatment

The GP registrar at a large practice in inner London decided to carry out, with the CCG pharmacy advisor, a small study looking at how many patients could switch their lipid-lowering medication from more costly preparations to simvastatin. A search was carried out and a plan devised involving the patients.

Although most patients were happy to change, some were not and the change was not made. For three patients the registrar had to liaise with the hospital specialists about the best course of action (a cardiologist and a lipid-specialist).

Two patients who were taking atorvastatin and rosuvastatin respectively could not be contacted. Both patients (a middle-aged male and a young female) were HIV-positive and on ART, including a protease inhibitor and a non-nucleoside inhibitor. They were looked after by different HIV-specialist centres in London. There had been correspondence from their

HIV specialists in the past, but no letters had been received in the past year. In both cases there had been no detailed information about their lipid levels although the correspondence noted 'hyperlipidaemia'.

While the practice was some way from automatically switching these last two patients from their present statin to simvastatin it is not difficult to see how this might have happened if staff had not been aware of the patients' HIV status. The study was therefore discussed in the practice's thrice-yearly critical incident seminar since it provided important information and key learning.

Learning points:
- Simvastatin is contraindicated for patients on some ART as the risk of a serious adverse event from drug interaction is extremely high.
- Any proposed change to long-term therapy should always be discussed with the patient and hospital specialist.

which may lead to clinical jaundice. This is harmless and only requires a change of regimen if the patient finds jaundice troublesome.

Other side effects caused by older antiretrovirals
- **Peripheral neuropathies**: painful or anaesthetic. They are mainly caused by didanosine and stavudine, less commonly lamivudine.
- **Bone marrow suppression** (anaemia, neutropenia) most commonly caused by zidovudine, stavudine and lamivudine.
- **Pancreatitis** was caused by didanosine, stavudine, abacavir and lamivudine.

Additional treatments for those with immunosuppression

Prophylaxis against opportunistic infections (OIs)

Pneumocystis pneumonia (PCP)

Patients who either have a CD4 count below 200 cells/μl or have already had an episode of PCP will be offered prophylaxis. Co-trimoxazole is the most effective agent although others are used. If the immune system recovers sufficiently following antiretroviral medication, this prophylaxis may be discontinued once the CD4 count is above 200 cells/μl and viral load is undetectable. Pentamidine nebulisers are used in the case of co-trimoxazole allergy.

Co-trimoxazole also protects against toxoplasmosis.

Mycobacterium avium intracellulare

Patients with a CD4 count below 50 cells/μl should be offered primary prophylaxis – usually azithromycin or rifabutin unless immune reconstitution is expected imminently.

Other OIs

Secondary prophylaxis is prescribed for some other OIs including cryptococcal disease, CMV and toxoplasmosis – these will be be stopped once durable immune reconstitution has been achieved.

The patient who will not attend for specialist care

Some patients with HIV drift out of or reject specialist care. There are several reasons why this might happen. The patient may have had a bad experience at a specialist unit or have encountered adverse effects of ART. They may be feeling better and believe that treatment is no longer needed. Sometimes overriding socio-economic or emotional problems have got in the way of attendance. They may hold cultural or religious beliefs regarding disease causation and conventional medicine. Finally HIV-related stigma in their community may be so pervasive that people may prefer to risk death than be seen coming out of an HIV clinic.

For more on stigma see page 88

If the GP has managed to keep a continuing relationship with the patient, this can be quite a stressful situation. The patient may not respond to discussion about the benefits of specialist care (with or without ART) and the need to attend. The GP should:

- confirm for themselves that the patient has the capacity to make decisions
- try to maintain their relationship and contact with the patient – this is sometimes the most they can achieve for some time

- explore exactly what the patient's reasons are for not wishing to attend the HIV clinic – there may be a problem that can be addressed. In some areas there is more than one local HIV clinic to which the patient could be referred if there are concerns around confidentiality or being recognised – or indeed the patient may be prepared to travel.
- continue to give gentle reminders to the patient of the health benefits of specialist care – whilst trying not to jeopardise the GP-patient relationship
- consider arranging (after discussion with the patient and the local lab) a CD4 count to assess how damaged their immunity is. With a high CD4 count the GP can be a bit more relaxed with the patient about the need for hospital review
- discuss the possibility of prophylactic treatments (such co-trimoxazole for PCP for those with a CD4 below 200/µl) with those that may not accept ART
- provide support to the patient's partner (if registered with you).

It is important to make sure you are fully aware of your responsibilities and what the GMC advises regarding patients who refuse specialist treatment. Always discuss the matter with your colleagues, and also seek advice about this from your medical defence union.

The dying patient

The advent of ART has meant that death as a result of HIV infection has become uncommon. Usually it occurs in those who present with advanced disease or who are affected by other disease processes. Nevertheless, deaths still occur and the primary care team is likely to be involved in decisions regarding care as death approaches. With ART it is harder to define when a patient is terminally ill, because, given time, there can be recovery of immunity following changes in choice of antiretroviral. However, the patient remains vulnerable to overwhelming infection until that happens. With this uncertainty about outcome, there is a need to integrate palliative and curative approaches to care, and the goals of HIV palliative care need to be redefined.

1. Planning care and advance decisions

See BMA (2007) *Advance decisions and proxy decision-making in medical treatment and research*

Several life-threatening episodes may occur before the final terminal event. So, if not already addressed, planning should begin early on after immunity has started to deteriorate.

People with HIV commonly want to be in control of their care and treatment. All should be helped, if necessary, to express their requirements and preferences, which may change depending on the type of illness or stage of the condition. The desire for maximum patient choice in matters of care and treatment is nowhere more important than during episodes of acute, potentially life-threatening illness or when the patient is clearly approaching the terminal phase. Wherever possible, dying patients should be able to have partner, family, friends and people they trust around them, as well as appropriate medical, nursing and social care.

A well-planned death can also help those left behind to cope with their loss. In the UK, living wills or advance directives were largely developed by and for people with AIDS, though they are now used more widely. GPs may be asked to look at such documents, or contribute to their contents. In such circumstances it is always advisable to seek further advice and guidance, for example the BMA's ethical guidance.

2. Involvement of other healthcare professionals

Although the course of advanced HIV disease may be more 'up and down' than other conditions requiring palliative care, GPs should still be able to draw on their experience. Continuity and communication are extremely important in palliative care, and general practice is well suited to providing these. The patient should be offered the support and involvement of palliative services and community nursing if appropriate. Some GPs can harness the support of specialist community nurses in HIV care. Hospice care may be needed. Respite care and symptom control are currently the most important indications for admission.

3. Wills

People with deteriorating immunity should be advised to make a will as a matter of priority to avoid distressing disagreements and resentment after death. Civil partnership and same-sex marriage legislation provides full legal recognition for gay partners. However, regardless of such legislation, the will and testament is the document recognised by law and, if in doubt, patients should be advised to seek legal advice.

4. Death certification

See GMC
Confidentiality
guidance:
Disclosure after a
patient's death

Death certification for people who have died of an HIV-related illness is really no different from that for death from other causes. If the clinician knows that the deceased has died from an HIV-related illness then this needs to be stated on the death certificate. It is still the case that confidentiality continues after death and in circumstances where the family do not know about their relative's HIV status, the situation needs sensitive handling, preferably by senior clinical staff. The guidance for the clinician completing the death certificate is clear and unambiguous – and this remains a legal requirement (see GMC guidance).

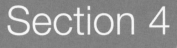

Section 4

HIV and the practice team

IN THIS SECTION

HIV and the practice team

Here we discuss the ways in which team members can play a key role in HIV prevention, and also in chronic disease management for those living with HIV.

GPs and practice nurses are excellently placed to support patients in the clinical management, and self-management, of this chronic condition.

We are familiar with approaches to support adherence and also to motivate for healthy lifestyle choices. GPs are experienced in the management of co-morbidities and polypharmacy. Practice policies (eg on confidentiality) and practice systems (such as active recall and reminders for immunisation) also support high quality care.

Sexual health promotion and HIV prevention in the practice

Practice teams can play an active part in promoting sexual health and reducing HIV transmission. For this role, clinical workers in primary care need both factual information and skills in sexual history taking and risk assessment.

For more, see BASHH/MEDFASH (2014) *Standards for the management of sexually transmitted infections (STIs)*

The British Association for Sexual Health and HIV and MEDFASH *Standards for the management of sexually transmitted infections (STIs)* provide clear guidance for all services that manage STIs. Standard 2, Clinical assessment, covers the need for appropriate history taking and Standard 7, Appropriately trained staff, covers competence and training.

Lack of knowledge about HIV, including a lack of understanding as to how it is transmitted or what constitutes risk, means that many of those who are at risk have not tested. This is why it is important for doctors, nurses and (particularly where prevalence of HIV is high) healthcare assistants to routinely discuss HIV and offer tests.

Practice nurses and GPs have opportunities to:
- discuss and assess risk of having or acquiring HIV with individual patients
- promote safer sexual practices and condom use with those who are or may be at risk
- promote HIV testing when appropriate

- promote hepatitis B testing and immunisation when appropriate
- support harm minimisation with injecting drug users.

Sexual health promotion interventions may occur during:
- travel advice consultations
- new patient checks
- contraceptive care
- cervical screening.

Post-exposure prophylaxis following sexual exposure (PEPSE)

For more on dealing with sexual assault, see BASHH (2011, updated 2012) *UK National Guidelines on the Management of Adult and Adolescent Complainants of Sexual Assault*

PEPSE is the emergency use of ART to prevent infection after exposure to high risk of sexual transmission of HIV. For example, it may be offered (depending on the treatment status of the source) to the uninfected sexual partner of someone known to have HIV in order to prevent infection after unprotected sex (such as when a condom has broken). It is also sometimes offered to individuals who have had unprotected sex with someone from a high-risk group but whose HIV status is unknown. Victims of sexual assault may also be offered PEPSE, depending on the risk assessment.

It is only recommended when the individual presents within 72 hours of exposure, and should be given as early as possible within this time frame, ideally no more than 24 hours after exposure.

PEPSE is available from HIV and GUM clinics and from Emergency Departments. Anyone presenting to primary care for PEPSE needs to be referred without delay to a specialist service where they can be assessed according to British Association for Sexual Health and HIV guidelines.

Pre-exposure prophylaxis

Pre-exposure prophylaxis (PrEP), taking HIV drugs before and after a possible exposure, is not available on the NHS at time of writing but can be accessed privately or via online generics services. Individuals taking PrEP should have regular STI screens, and some medication regimens require monitoring of renal function. Clinicians should be aware as this may have implications for drug interactions (see www.hiv-druginteractions.org).

Familiar – and diverse – needs amongst those with HIV

GPs and practice nurses are well placed to work with a wide range of people as they know their practice populations well. HIV can affect and infect anyone, but in the UK it is still most common in certain population groups. These are:
- men who have sex with men
- people from countries of high HIV prevalence especially Sub-Saharan

Africa, but increasingly other areas, including the Caribbean and Eastern Europe

- injecting drug users.

Social exclusion and disadvantage can make people more vulnerable to HIV, which is over represented amongst, for example, prisoners, the homeless and asylum seekers.

For PEP following occupational exposure see page 94

1. HIV stigma – still a real issue

Members of all these groups may already feel marginalised or stigmatised in UK society and this can be exacerbated by the stigma and discrimination associated with HIV. Practitioners in primary healthcare need to be aware of some of the emotional and social pressures on people in these groups.

In some communities, HIV infection is still widely thought to be incurable and people are afraid of contracting it. The link between sex or drug injecting and illness means that people who contract HIV are often thought to have brought it upon themselves as a result of personal irresponsibility or immorality. These factors combine to create a stigma that underpins prejudice, discrimination and even violence towards people with HIV.

The impact of stigma

Stigma leads to some people not seeking HIV testing or being reluctant to agree to an HIV test, despite knowing they might be at risk.

Few people with HIV feel able to be completely open about their status. A significant number do not tell employers or work colleagues or even close family members and friends. Some do not feel able to confide in their sexual partners or spouses for fear of rejection or abuse. The isolation and fear of being 'found out' and of possible rejection or discrimination, can lead to stress and depression.

Sometimes these fears are unfounded and confiding in trusted family members and friends can provide great support, but not always. Pregnant women have been subjected to physical violence, evicted from shared homes and ostracised by their communities when discovered to have HIV.

Some think that stigma and discrimination have gone away, but unfortunately they have not. Being aware of this as a clinician can only help

Support against stigma and discrimination

For more, see NAM (2012) *HIV stigma and discrimination*

People with HIV are now covered from the point of diagnosis by the provisions of the Equality Act 2010. This offers protection against discrimination in a variety of fields, including employment and the provision of goods, facilities and services. Voluntary and community organisations which provide support and services for people with HIV have helped many to cope with both the medical and social consequences of a positive HIV diagnosis.

2. Men who have sex with men (MSM)

This term is used to include both men who identify as homosexual (and may call themselves gay) and those who have sexual encounters with other men without considering themselves to be homosexual. Gay men may have a sense of belonging and access to gay-oriented culture. However, other men who have sex with men often see themselves as bisexual or even heterosexual, are sometimes married, and may not be open about their same-sex encounters.

If a gay patient has a long-term partner, they too may well be registered at the practice. In these circumstances the team can play a supportive role, particularly if the partner has needs (as a carer, for example). Civil partnerships and same-sex marriage provide same-sex couples with the same rights as heterosexual married couples, including next-of-kin status.

3. Migrants from areas of high HIV prevalence

The prevalence of HIV in peoples' countries of origin is reflected in their communities in the UK. Thus the prevalence of HIV amongst people from Sub-Saharan Africa, in particular, or parts of the Caribbean, Far East and Eastern Europe are higher, sometimes much higher, than the UK average (figure 7). In some cultures, HIV-related fear and prejudice can be strong, with resultant stigma and secrecy. Many people from high prevalence

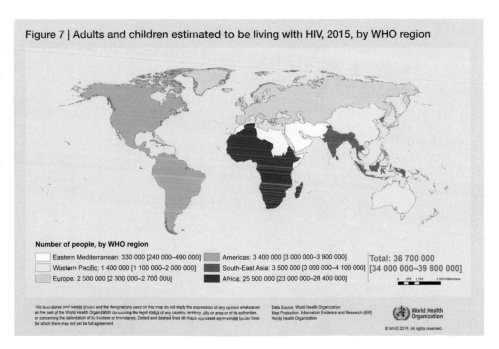

Figure 7 | Adults and children estimated to be living with HIV, 2015, by WHO region

Number of people, by WHO region

Eastern Mediterranean: 330 000 [240 000–490 000]	Americas: 3 400 000 [3 000 000–3 900 000]	Total: 36 700 000
Western Pacific: 1 400 000 [1 100 000–2 000 000]	South-East Asia: 3 500 000 [3 000 000–4 100 000]	[34 000 000–39 800 000]
Europe: 2 500 000 [2 300 000–2 700 000]	Africa: 25 500 000 [23 000 000–28 400 000]	

countries will know of family members or friends who are living with, or have died from, HIV. However, there may be a great reluctance to acknowledge this openly due to stigma. HIV may affect both parents as well as the children (infected or not), creating major family needs. Diagnosis in an adult should prompt consideration of possible infection in their children, who may have been born in a country not systematically intervening to prevent mother-to-child transmission.

Cultural and religious beliefs may affect how people cope with a diagnosis of HIV and their beliefs about illness and treatment. It is important to present information in a culturally sensitive way and check patients' understanding – it has been known for people with limited English to hear 'the result is positive' as meaning that they are not infected with HIV. Beliefs should be explored in an open and non-judgemental manner (if not always in the first consultation, when the diagnosis is given) as they may affect future adherence to treatment. Have patient information leaflets about HIV available and give contact details of local support groups and HIV services. The GP's knowledge of the local community helps in providing a focus of care for families affected by HIV.

In many of the countries in these areas, attitudes to homosexuality are hostile and some have laws which criminalise sex between men. Men from these areas may therefore be less likely than those from the UK to disclose sexual activity with other men.

Some people with HIV are asylum seekers or refugees who have lost family members to violence and have fled their country. Some asylum seekers may ultimately be returned to countries where HIV treatment is unavailable to them.

Worries about employment, immigration or asylum can compound anxiety about confidentiality and disclosure of HIV status. When finding interpreters, it is important to be aware of HIV stigma and concerns about confidentiality within their community.

4. Substance misuse

Injecting drug use

For more, see the Substance misuse management in general practice website (SMMGP), www.smmgp.org.uk

Those who have acquired HIV through injecting drugs (even if they no longer use them) may be aware of a double stigma – as drug users they are a socially excluded group, and this may be compounded by their HIV status. Those who have not wished, or been unable, to access support may be locked in a cycle of problems connected to their drug use. Dependent drug use may restrict the ability to attend appointments or take medication regularly. For some, HIV may not be a priority in the face of the daily problems associated with drug dependence. Low self-esteem, being in prison, previous abuse and other psycho-emotional problems are often underlying issues.

GPs involved in appropriate substitute prescribing in primary care will be aware of the benefits of this for the patient, in terms of harm reduction and access to healthcare. Do not assume that all injecting drug users are fully aware of the risks of sharing equipment or using non-sterile needles. It does no harm to explore their understanding and reinforce advice.

Injecting is also a risk for some groups who would not be perceived as typical drug users, such as those who inject anabolic steroids and tanning drugs.

Recreational drugs and alcohol
A range of substances can be associated with risky sexual behaviour, such as alcohol and a number of non-opioid drugs used by, for example, young people, clubbers and men who have sex with men (MSM). There is growing concern about the use of such drugs by some MSM specifically to facilitate sex (so called chemsex), with higher sexual risk-taking. Injecting is also increasing within this group, often with little knowledge of the risks, resulting in high levels of equipment-sharing.

Dependency on drugs or alcohol should be managed in the usual way. As is usual, underlying mental health difficulties such as social anxiety, depression or low self-esteem may exacerbate these problems

5. Support organisations
There may be organisations offering support to MSM, Africans or other migrants with HIV infection in your area – your patient may (or may not) wish to be put in touch. Local organisations offering support to drug users may provide specific services for those with or at risk of HIV.

Practice policies and systems

1. Ensuring confidentiality and avoiding discrimination
Some patients with HIV perceive negative attitudes towards them from some GPs or other members of the primary care team. Many have fears relating to confidentiality, especially around sensitive information such as HIV status, sexual orientation or lifestyle. Fear of breach of confidentiality is one of the main reasons patients with HIV cite when deciding whether or not to allow the hospital to communicate with their GP.

Developing a practice that is alive to patient concerns about confidentiality and fears of discrimination will support:
* open discussion of, and testing for, HIV with those who may be at risk
* disclosure of HIV status by those who already know they are infected
* open discussion about safer sexual and injecting practices
* improved quality of care for people with HIV infection.

Several studies have shown that the following interventions help in allaying the fears of patients:

- ensuring that your practitioners and clinicians are non-judgmental and empathic to different lifestyles. Consider in-house training for the team
- developing and implementing a non-discrimination policy with your practice – then displaying it to your patients
- developing and implementing an appropriate confidentiality statement – then displaying it to your patients.

(There are examples of these in the Sexual Health module of the e-GP programme)

Practices which gain a reputation for being 'HIV-friendly' may see an increase in registrations from people with HIV as they exercise their right to choose their GP and 'shop around' to find the right practice.

2. Systems and record keeping

To support HIV testing

For aide-memoire
see pages 96–97

For a clinician to request any investigation, verbal consent is needed and HIV is no different. A brief record entry is appropriate to indicate the test has been mentioned.

For the patient with HIV

For your patients with HIV, see National AIDS Trust (2014) *Confidentiality in the NHS: Your Information, Your Rights. A guide on how personal confidential information on HIV is stored, used and shared within the NHS in England*

Some patients will be anxious about how their HIV status is to be recorded in the practice. It is best to raise the subject so this issue can be addressed and the benefits outlined (as well as the risks if the diagnosis is not clearly recorded).

The use of computers

As with other conditions, there are different options for Read coding HIV infection. Having an agreed code for the team (or CCG) will of course support searches for patient care and follow-up (such as flu immunisation or annual cervical screening).

Computer screens should not be visible to anyone who is accompanying a patient, although in practice this may be difficult to achieve in a small consulting room.

Communication to support clinical care

The success of practice information systems depends on reliable and rapid communication to and from the hospital each time the patient has attended and also when significant test results become available. Historically HIV is one topic where communication with GPs has not been standard, although this continues to change. You can let the patient know that you are keen to be involved with their care – they can then help ensure the specialist sends you an update. Electronic transfer of information is making this much easier, much faster and more efficient.

Records of antiretroviral and other drugs

Even if drugs are prescribed solely by the hospital, a clear record should be kept on the patient medication list (as acute, rather than repeat, so patients cannot obtain them accidentally). This can help in avoiding key drug interactions by alerting clinicians to their use by the patient, thus enabling them to check with www.hiv-druginteractions.org. Automated drug interaction software is a bonus, but should not be relied upon alone, as it risks being less up to date than the specialised website.

Records of CD4 count and viral load

Computer systems enable a simple template to be set up for use with patients with HIV. The most recent blood results can then be entered when they are made available by the hospital, thus ensuring quick reference should a patient attend with symptoms.

Review date

A review date system can act as a reminder to check that records, notably the blood monitoring results, are up to date. It is better to spend time chasing an absent CD4 result before you are faced with a patient with a bad cough.

3. Health and safety

Hepatitis B immunisation

The practice should have a system to ensure that staff who handle clinical specimens are immune to hepatitis B.

Prevention of needlestick injuries

Universal precautions in handling sharp instruments and body fluids are essential to reduce the risk of contracting HIV or other blood-borne viral infections in the healthcare setting. Approved sterilisation procedures and adequate disposal of sharp instruments are crucial components of this process. It is easy to forget how much blood-borne infection is undiagnosed: assume that all patients are potentially infected.

IMPORTANT!
A 'high risk' needlestick injury requires rapid and decisive action. Ensure all team members are aware of the practice policy on PEP.

Management of needlestick injuries

A 'high risk' needlestick injury requires rapid and decisive action if post-exposure prophylaxis (PEP) is to be given in time. This should be as soon as possible after the injury (within hours) to maximise effectiveness.

Post-exposure prophylaxis for occupational exposure

Discuss, develop and implement a practice policy on PEP with guidance from local occupational health and/or virology and ensure all team members are aware of its existence. It is not good practice for the affected healthcare worker to have to organise their own care in this situation.

PEP policies in primary care should:
- advise how to manage the wound
- make clear the urgency and limited window of opportunity
- clarify who should be contacted for advice in your locality and how, including out of hours
- refer to locally agreed protocols for provision of PEP
- take into account other blood-borne viruses such as hepatitis B and C
- be adopted only in association with discussion and training.

PEP starter packs are usually held in the local hospital and, given the urgency, it is customary for PEP to be started and a thorough risk assessment to be made later. This allows for discontinuation where appropriate.

The HIV-infected healthcare worker

The majority of procedures carried out in the primary care setting (assuming appropriate infection control procedures) pose no risk of transmission of HIV from healthcare worker to patient. Employing people infected with HIV is generally not a risk as long as they are on effective ART – ie they have an undetectable viral load. For more details as to advice on testing and treatment for healthcare workers see the guidance produced by Public Health England.

See Public Health England (2014) *The Management of HIV infected Healthcare Workers who perform exposure prone procedures: updated guidance, January 2014*

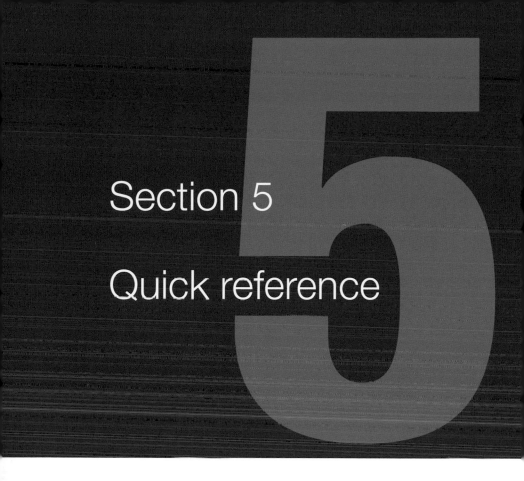

Section 5

Quick reference

IN THIS SECTION

Quick reference

HIV testing key points

Essentials
Make sure you explain:
- the benefits of testing and medical advantages of knowing one's HIV status
- how the patient will get the result.

Check their contact details
- Will the patient be given their result in an appointment, or by another means? Confirm the plan, including what the patient should do if they do not hear as expected (safety net).

Has the patient given clear consent to an HIV (or other) test?

Other areas to consider if needed
Does the patient understand:
- how HIV is transmitted?
- the difference between HIV and AIDS?
- the significance of the window period and the possible need for a repeat test?

Discussion of risk
- Risk to date, including drug and alcohol use affecting risk behaviour.
- Future risk/risk reduction

Discussion of implications of positive result

Discussion of implications of negative result
(ie as a wake-up call to change any risky behaviour)

Confidentiality

Coping with the wait
- Who knows they are having the test?
- Who is it safe to tell?

If the patient will be attending for their result, ask them not to drink alcohol or take recreational drugs on that day.

Other useful points to consider

- Is there any written information that should be given to the patient?
- Is the test best done in primary care?
- Should there be any associated tests (eg hepatitis B or C, syphilis, sickle screen, rubella etc)?
- Is a repeat test required to cover the window period?
- Does the patient have a supply of condoms/lubricant?

Antiretrovirals by group

This list centres on antiretrovirals currently in routine use and was correct at the time of writing. Up-to-date lists of agents are available on the following websites: www.bnf.org, www.hiv-druginteractions.org and http://i-base.info

Current antiretroviral drugs				
Nucleoside/tide reverse transcriptase inhibitors (NRTIs)	Non-nucleoside reverse transcriptase inhibitors (NNRTIs)	Protease inhibitors (PIs)	Entry inhibitors (EIs)	Integrase inhibitors (IIs)
abacavir	efavirenz	atazanavir (usually used with a boosting agent*)	enfuvirtide (T-20)	raltegravir
emtricitabine (FTC)	etravirine	darunavir (used with a boosting agent*)	maraviroc	elvitegravir (boosted* with cobicistat)
lamivudine (3TC)	nevirapine	lopinavir (boosted* with ritonavir)		dolutegravir
tenofovir DF (TDF)	rilpivirine	saquinavir (usually used with a boosting agent*)		
tenofovir alafenamide (TAF)				
zidovudine (AZT)				

* Boosting agents: currently two drugs (ritonavir and cobicistat are used to increase drug levels of antiretrovirals through their inhibitory actions on cytochrome P450 (CYPs) enzyme systems. Ritonavir is an antiretroviral in its own right, but poorly tolerated: it is used in smaller doses as a booster. Cobicistat is newer and is gaining favour because it acts more selectively and so has fewer additional drug interactions.

Examples of combination tablets	
Example trade name (prescribing switches to generics when patents expire)	**Contains**
Atripla	efavirenz, tenofovir DF, emtricitabine
Eviplera	rilpivirine, tenofovir DF, emtricitabine
Stribild	elvitegravir, cobicistat (booster), tenofovir DF, emtricitabine
Triumeq	dolutegravir, abacavir, lamivudine
Truvada	tenofovir DF, emtricitabine
Kivexa	abacavir, lamivudine
Descovy	tenofovir alafenamide, emtricitabine
Genvoya	tenofovir alafenamide, emtricitabine, elvitegravir, cobicistat (booster)
Odefsey	tenofovir alafenamide, emtricitabine, rilpivirine
Kaletra	lopinavir, ritonavir (booster)
Combivir	lamivudine, zidovudine
Trizivir	abacavir, lamivudine, zidovudine

Trade names are not often used in the UK for single drug tablets. They are used more commonly for combination tablets, examples of which are listed above. Trade names are all given in the BNF which is a good source for information on names and formulations, as the available combinations are rapidly changing.

Drug interactions – further information

Either
Check www.hiv-druginteractions.org – a very reliable, internationally recognised resource (with respect to drug interactions this is more comprehensive and more regularly updated than the BNF)
Or
Check the Summary of Product Characteristics for the antiretroviral drug(s) in question at www.medicines.org.uk
Or
Contact a specialist HIV pharmacist for advice – there may be one at your local HIV clinic.

Drug side effects

The table below describes some of the commoner and more important side effects of antiretrovirals. Contact an HIV specialist if you are uncertain as to the cause of your patient's symptoms.

Side effect	NRTI	NNRTI	PI	EIs	IIs
Hypersensitivity	abacavir	nevirapine			dolutegravir
Central nervous system toxicities					
• Mood disturbance		possibly all but most pronounced with efavirenz	psychosis possible with all – very rare		dolutegravir
• Insomnia		efavirenz			dolutegravir
Hyperlipidaemia	older agents only	efavirenz	all, but less likely with atazanavir		
Lipoatrophy/ lipodystrophy	older agents only	possibly all	possibly all		
Diabetes (type II)	older agents only	possibly all	possibly all		
Renal problems	tenofovir DF				
Ureteric colic, renal and ureteric stones			atazanavir indinavir		
Hepatic toxicity	possible with all	Greatest risk nevirapine Possible with all	darunavir tipranavir when boosted with ritonavir		
• Jaundice			atazanavir		
Bone marrow suppression	older agents only				
Pancreatitis	didanosine stavudine (rare) abacavir (rare) lamivudine (rare)				

A guide to managing HIV-related problems

A patient with HIV who presents with any symptoms might have:
- problems which relate to HIV disease (check the most recent CD4 count)
- side effects of ART
- a health problem completely unrelated to HIV.

Patients who have developed symptoms which relate to HIV disease might have stopped taking their medication (ask) or might have developed resistance to their ART regimen. Current CD4 counts and viral load will clarify.

For patients who have not started ART, most of the problems mentioned below will improve, become less severe and rarely occur once they are established on ART.

Seek advice from an HIV specialist if any of the conditions below are severe or resistant to treatment.

It is important to be aware of possible ART interactions with all medication including inhalers, nasal sprays and injections, see www.hiv-druginteractions.org

Constitutional symptoms		
Condition	Notes	Management
Night sweats	Exclude serious causes, eg lymphoma, TB, chronic gut infection. Always consider menopause in women (HIV may be associated with earlier menopause).	Supportive management.
Fatigue	Exclude serious causes eg tumour or opportunistic infections. Exclude common causes: • anaemia • thyroid deficiency • vitamin B deficiency • testosterone deficiency. Test for calcium, renal function. TFTs, FBC in all. Consider ART side effects. Consider viral hepatitis.	May be managed in secondary or primary care, depending on cause. Testosterone replacement sometimes used if deficiency confirmed, seek specialist advice.
Weight loss	Exclude serious causes (tumour, chronic infection, opportunistic infections).	Dietary supplementation may have a role if all potentially serious causes have been excluded.

Skin conditions		
Condition	**Notes**	**Management**
Fungal infections		Generally respond to topical antifungals (often combined with topical steroids). Prolonged or repeated treatment may be required. Oral antifungals may be indicated for some (esp. nail infections).
Herpes zoster Herpes simplex		Will respond to antivirals such as aciclovir but longer courses at higher doses may be needed. Long-term use of antivirals is helpful if the problem is recurrent.
Warts Molluscum contagiosum		Topical imiquimod or podophyllotoxin. Cryotherapy.
Bacterial infections eg impetigo folliculitis		Oral antibiotics are more effective and less likely to be associated with resistance than topical antibiotics.
Seborrhoeic dermatitis		Topical antifungal and hydrocortisone combinations. Antifungal shampoos often helpful.
Psoriasis		Usual management, but may be much less responsive.
Kaposi's sarcoma		Usually improves on ART, may require specialist treatment.

The mouth		
Condition	**Notes**	**Management**
Oral candida	Can cause significant discomfort and difficulty in eating/drinking.	Systemic anti-fungal agents are effective. If recurrent can indicate poor immune function and need for specialist opinion. Long-term use of antifungals occasionally indicated if the problem is recurrent. May need referral if severe or resistant infection.
Aphthous ulceration		Topical oral steroid creams. Specialists use thalidomide if troublesome.
Oral hairy leukoplakia		Generally asymptomatic and does not require treatment.
Gingivitis	Maintaining good oral hygiene and dental care is important for all immunocompromised patients.	Chlorhexidine mouth washes. Oral metronidazole. Referral to dentist.
Kaposi's sarcoma		Requires specialist treatment. May disappear with effective ART.
Dental abscess		Oral antibiotics. Referral to dentist.

The rest of the gastrointestinal tract		
Condition	**Notes**	**Management**
Nausea	May be caused by ART.	Managed with either a dopaminergic agent (domperidone) or agents such as levomepromazine.
Oesophageal candida	Indicates severe immunosuppression.	As for oral candida (see The mouth above) but generally managed by specialists or GPwSI as usually diagnosed at endoscopy.
Diarrhoea	Possible causes: • side effect of ART • pancreatic insufficiency • HIV in the intestinal mucosa • intestinal pathogens Check if could be travel-related diarrhoea. Take stool samples. More likely to have lactose intolerance and remember coeliac too.	Management should be guided by microscopy and culture results and information on drug interactions: seek specialist advice if necessary. Loperamide for symptomatic treatment. Codeine is sometimes helpful. Salmonella and campylobacter respond to ciprofloxacin or macrolides as appropriate. Less common organisms such as *Cryptosporidium* sp and *Microsporidium* sp may be responsible if patient has a low CD4 count. Check faecal calprotectin. Consider trial of Creon (pancrelipase) if pancreatic insufficiency suspected (may need high dose).

Respiratory conditions		
Condition	**Notes**	**Management**
Chest infection	Exclude PCP (see pages 31–32). Exclude TB-like infections (see page 33).	Community-acquired chest infections should respond to first line antibiotics.

Neurological conditions – see also page 34 for serious conditions that require admission		
Condition	**Notes**	**Management**
Peripheral neuropathy	May be caused by HIV or antiretrovirals.	Pain management similar to usual approaches to neuropathic pain. Gabapentin or other drugs used in neuralgia may help.

Genital conditions

Condition	Notes	Management
Genital candida		Topical or systemic antifungal agents (clotrimazole, fluconazole). Systemic antifungals are sometimes used long-term to prevent recurrence.
Genital herpes		Aciclovir – may be needed in longer courses and at a higher end of the dose range than usual. Long-term use of aciclovir or similar may be used to suppress frequent recurrences.
Genital and perianal warts		Frequently recurrent and more difficult to treat. Topical therapy (imiquimod or podophyllotoxin) or cryotherapy may help. Refer to GUM unless responding well to topical therapy. Anal intraepithelial neoplasms and anal squamous cell carcinomas are much more common in the HIV positive population so referral for anoscopy is indicated if there are atypical features.

Sexual dysfunction

Condition	Notes	Management
Erectile dysfunction Loss of libido	May be multifactorial. HIV-related causes include: • effect of HIV • fear of transmitting infection • ART • vascular problems. In men check testosterone level.	Phosphodiesterase inhibitors can be used, but they interact with PIs and NNRTIs and expert advice should be sought. Testosterone replacement is sometimes used on specialist advice. There is increasing evidence that erectile dysfunction can predict underlying vascular problems and hence increased risk for CVD/ischaemic heart disease.

Psychological conditions		
Condition	Notes	Management
Stress	Stress is common. May be exacerbated by stigma.	Supportive counselling and/or specialist or psychological support is sometimes necessary.
Depression Bipolar disorder	May be seen more commonly in people with HIV. Some antiretrovirals may be associated with psychiatric disturbance.	Beware drug interactions if considering antidepressants, especially citalopram.
HIV-related brain impairment	Can cause functional impairment and lead to significant care needs.	Seek specialist advice. Consider needs of carer(s).

Visual problems
See page 35 for CMV retinitis, a serious condition that requires urgent referral to ophthalmology.

Information to support implementation of UK HIV testing guidelines

Clinical indicator diseases for HIV infection

UK and European guidelines recommend offering an HIV test to every patient presenting with a clinical indicator disease for HIV infection. (See table)

Definitions of indicator conditions and recommendations for HIV testing

1. Conditions which are AIDS defining among people living with HIV*

Strongly recommend testing

Neoplasms
- Cervical cancer
- Non-Hodgkin lymphoma
- Kaposi's sarcoma

Bacterial infections
- *Mycobacterium tuberculosis*, pulmonary or extrapulmonary
- *Mycobacterium avium* complex (MAC) or *Mycobacterium kansasii*, disseminated or extrapulmonary
- Mycobacterium, other species or unidentified species, disseminated or extrapulmonary
- Pneumonia, recurrent (2 or more episodes in 12 months)
- Salmonella septicaemia, recurrent

Viral infections
- Cytomegalovirus retinitis
- Cytomegalovirus, other (except liver, spleen, glands)
- Herpes simplex, ulcer(s) > 1 month, bronchitis/pneumonitis
- Progressive multifocal leucoencephalopathy

Parasitic infections
- Cerebral toxoplasmosis
- Cryptosporidiosis diarrhoea, > 1 month
- Isosporiasis, > 1 month
- Atypical disseminated leishmaniasis
- Reactivation of American trypanosomiasis (meningoencephalitis or myocarditis)

Fungal infections
- *Pneumocystis* pneumonia (PCP)
- Candidiasis, oesophageal
- Candidiasis, bronchial/tracheal/lungs
- Cryptococcosis, extrapulmonary
- Histoplasmosis, disseminated/extrapulmonary
- Coccidioidomycosis, disseminated/extrapulmonary
- Penicilliosis, disseminated

2a. Conditions associated with an undiagnosed HIV prevalence of ≥ 0.1%

Strongly recommend testing

- Sexually transmitted infections
- Malignant lymphoma
- Anal cancer/dysplasia
- Cervical dysplasia
- Herpes zoster
- Hepatitis B or C (acute or chronic)
- Mononucleosis-like illness
- Unexplained leukocytopenia/thrombocytopenia lasting > 4 weeks
- Seborrhoeic dermatitis/exanthema
- Invasive pneumococcal disease
- Unexplained fever
- Candidaemia
- Visceral leishmaniasis
- Pregnancy (implications for the unborn child)**

2b. Other conditions considered likely to have an undiagnosed HIV prevalence of > 0.1%

Offer testing

- Primary lung cancer
- Lymphocytic meningitis
- Oral hairy leukoplakia
- Severe or atypical psoriasis
- Guillain-Barré syndrome
- Mononeuritis
- Subcortical dementia
- Multiple sclerosis-like disease
- Peripheral neuropathy
- Unexplained weight loss
- Unexplained lymphadenopathy
- Unexplained oral candidiasis
- Unexplained chronic diarrhoea
- Unexplained chronic renal impairment
- Hepatitis A
- Community-acquired pneumonia
- Candidiasis

3. Conditions where not identifying the presence of HIV infection may have significant adverse implications for the individual's clinical management

Offer testing

- Conditions requiring aggressive immuno-suppressive therapy:
  - Cancer
  - Transplantation
  - Auto-immune disease treated with immunosuppressive therapy
- Primary space occupying lesion of the brain
- Idiopathic/thrombotic thrombocytopenic purpura

---

* Based on Centers for Disease Control and Prevention (CDC) and World Health Organization (WHO) classification system.

** Pregnancy is included in the 'strongly recommended' category because antenatal HIV testing is essential for prevention of mother-to-child transmission.

HIV in Europe, *HIV Indicator Conditions: Guidance for Implementing HIV Testing in Adults in Health Care Settings*. October 2012, updated 2016.

Local diagnosed HIV prevalence

The *UK National Guidelines for HIV Testing 2008* suggest an HIV test should be routinely offered as part of new patient checks in general practice and for hospital admissions, where local diagnosed HIV prevalence is high (currently defined as over two per 1,000 population aged 15–59 years). NICE guidance for England (being updated in 2016) supports this and also recommends that, in such areas, general practice should offer and recommend an HIV test to anyone who is undergoing a blood test for another reason.

UK data tables, including *HIV prevalence by Local Authority of residence* in England, can be found on the PHE website (www.gov.uk/government/statistics/hiv-annual-data-tables). Comparative data for England in different formats can also be found in PHE's *Sexual and Reproductive Health Profiles* (http://fingertips.phe.org.uk/profile/sexualhealth).

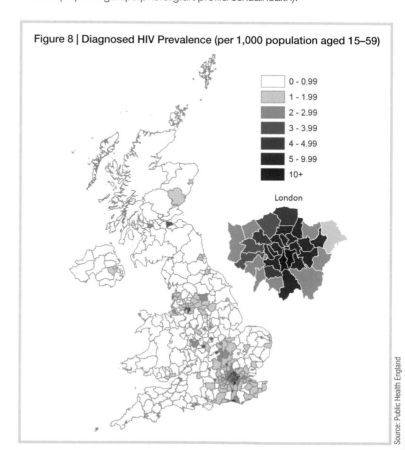

Figure 8 | Diagnosed HIV Prevalence (per 1,000 population aged 15–59)

	0 - 0.99
	1 - 1.99
	2 - 2.99
	3 - 3.99
	4 - 4.99
	5 - 9.99
	10+

London

Source: Public Health England

Useful organisations and websites

aidsmap
www.aidsmap.com
Extensive information on treatments and the latest research. Database of HIV organisations worldwide (including UK). Leaflets for patients available to download or order and some online information resources in French, Portuguese, Spanish, Romanian and Russian.

British Association for Sexual Health and HIV (BASHH)
www.bashh.org
Specialist society for professionals in GUM/HIV. Produces standards and clinical effectiveness guidelines and runs training on STIs and HIV.

British HIV Association (BHIVA)
www.bhiva.org
Regularly updated guidelines for all aspects of HIV treatment and care and twice yearly conferences.

Children's HIV Association of the UK and Ireland (CHIVA)
www.chiva.org.uk
Guidelines on treatment and care of HIV-infected children, plus resources for health and social care professionals, parents and young people.

HIV i-Base
http://i-base.info/
Treatment activist group providing technical and non-technical bulletins and guides to HIV treatment and a Q&A service (by phone, email and online)

HIV Pharmacy Association (HIVPA)
www.hivpa.org/patient-information-leaflets/
Professional organisation for specialist HIV pharmacists. Patient information leaflets for individual antiretroviral drugs available online for non-members.

HIV TIPs (HIV testing in practice)
www.medfash.org.uk/hiv-tips
Online educational tool from MEDFASH to help increase HIV testing in general practice. Contains materials for individual and team learning.

HIV Drug Interactions
www.hiv-druginteractions.org
Comprehensive listings of interactions between HIV drugs and others, including herbal medicines and recreational drugs, provided by the

University of Liverpool Pharmacology Research Labs. They will answer
individual queries from doctors.

National AIDS Trust
www.nat.org.uk
A national policy organisation. Useful information on legal and policy
issues for people with HIV and professionals.

Public Health England
www.gov.uk/government/collections/hiv-surveillance-data-and-
management
Up-to-date figures for HIV and other infections in the UK, including graphs
and slides that can be downloaded.
http://fingertips.phe.org.uk/profile/sexualhealth
Interactive maps, charts and tables on sexual and reproductive health
including HIV.

Scottish HIV and AIDS Group (SHIVAG)
www.shivag.co.uk
Professional website with news, discussion forums and useful documents
regarding HIV in Scotland.

Substance misuse management in general practice (SMMGP)
www.smmgp.org.uk
Organisation providing information and support to GPs prescribing for
drug users. Produces a regular newsletter.

Information for patients

Leaflets to have in the practice

You may wish to browse some of the websites above to find suitable
leaflets for your patients. Below are two initial suggestions. Many leaflets
are now available as either free downloads or printed versions for which
there may be a charge.

HIV FPA
www.fpa.org.uk/product/hiv-sexually-transmitted-infections-
booklets#product-content
An information leaflet about HIV and HIV testing for the general public.
A range of leaflets on other STIs is also available from FPA.

Your Next Steps NAM
www.aidsmap.com/Your-next-steps/page/1412486/
This booklet is for people who have just found out they have HIV. A range
of other booklets for people living with HIV is also available from NAM.

Support services

You may well have local organisations working with people with HIV. Here
we list just a few national organisations which may help you or your
patient to identify local ones.

Terrence Higgins Trust
www.tht.org.uk
The largest voluntary sector provider of HIV and sexual health services in
the UK, with centres in many British towns and cities. Also produces a
wide range of online and printed resources on living with HIV, HIV
prevention and sexual health.
THT Direct helpline: 0808 802 1221

Positively UK
www.positivelyuk.org
Provides peer-led support, advocacy and information to women, men and
young people living with HIV to manage any aspect of their diagnosis,
care and life with HIV.
Helpline answered by people living with HIV: 020 7713 0444

Sexual Health Line England
www.patient.info/support/sexual-health-line-england
Helpline: 0300 123 7123
Free confidential helpline for anyone concerned about HIV or sexual
health. Translation services available and can provide details of local HIV
organisations.

Sexual Health Scotland
www.sexualhealthscotland.co.uk
Information on sexual health and HIV, including listing of sources of help in
Scotland and sexual health service finder.
General information line: 0800 22 44 88

Positive Life (Northern Ireland)
www.positivelifeni.com
Voluntary organisation offering a range of services and support across
Northern Ireland for people living with and affected by HIV.

Professional development for clinicians on HIV and sexual health

A range of options for face-to-face and online education about HIV, sexual health and HIV-associated conditions is available from:

e-GP
www.e-lfh.org.uk/programmes/general-practitioners

Royal College of General Practitioners (RCGP)
www.rcgp.org.uk

British Association for Sexual Health and HIV (BASHH)
www.bashh.org

Faculty of Sexual and Reproductive Healthcare (FSRH)
www.fsrh.org

BMJ Learning
www.learning.bmj.com/learning

Key articles

HIV testing

Hsu DT, Ruf M, O'Shea S et al (2013) Diagnosing HIV infection in patients presenting with glandular fever-like illness in primary care: are we missing primary HIV infection? HIV Med 14(1):60-3.
www.onlinelibrary.wiley.com/doi/10.1111/j.1468-1293.2012.01023.x/full

Leber W, McMullen H, Anderson J et al (2015) Promotion of rapid testing for HIV in primary care (RHIVA2): a cluster-randomised controlled trial. *Lancet HIV* 2:229–235
www.thelancet.com/journals/lanhiv/article/PIIS2352-3018(15)00059-4/abstract

Sullivan AK, Raben D, Reekie J et al. (2013) Feasibility and effectiveness of indicator condition-guided testing for HIV: Results from HIDES I (HIV Indicator Diseases across Europe Study). *PLoS One* 2013;8(1):e52845.
www.journals.plos.org/plosone/article?id=10.1371/journal.pone.0052845

Benefits of early antiretroviral therapy

Cohen MS, Chen YQ, McCauley M et al (2011) Prevention of HIV-1 infection with early antiretroviral therapy. *N Engl J Med* 365: 493–505.
www.nejm.org/doi/full/10.1056/NEJMoa1105243#t=article

Ping L-H, Jabara CB, Rodrigo AG et al (2013) HIV-1 transmission during early antiretroviral therapy: evaluation of two HIV-1 transmission events in the HPTN 052 prevention study. *PLoS ONE* 8(9): e71557
www.journals.plos.org/plosone/article?id=10.1371/journal.pone.0071557

The INSIGHT START Study Group (2015) Initiation of antiretroviral therapy in early asymptomatic HIV infection. *N Engl J Med* 373:795-807.
www.nejm.org/doi/full/10.1056/NEJMoa1506816#t=article

Effectiveness of HIV pre-exposure prophylaxis

McCormack S, Dunn DT, Desai M et al (2016) Pre-exposure prophylaxis to prevent the acquisition of HIV-1 infection (PROUD): effectiveness results from the pilot phase of a pragmatic open-label randomized trial. *The Lancet* 387:53-60.
www.thelancet.com/journals/lancet/article/PIIS0140-6736(15)00056-2/abstract

Bibliography

This bibliography provides details of the publications referred to in this booklet.

Association of British Insurers & British Medical Association *GP report insurance package.*
www.bma.org.uk/advice/employment/ethics/confidentiality-and-health-records/gp-report-insurance-package

British Association for Sexual Health and HIV and Expert Advisory Group on AIDS (2014) *BASHH/EAGA Statement on HIV window period.*
www.gov.uk/government/publications/time-period-for-hiv-testing-position-statement

British Association for Sexual Health and HIV (2012) *UK National Guidelines on the Management of Adult and Adolescent Complainants of Sexual Assault 2011 (updated 2012).*
www.bashh.org/documents/4450.pdf

British Association for Sexual Health and HIV (2015) *UK Guideline for the use of HIV Post-Exposure Prophylaxis Following Sexual Exposure (PEPSE) 2015.*
www.bashh.org/documents/PEPSE%202015.pdf

British Association for Sexual Health and HIV, British HIV Association, British Infection Society (2008) *UK National Guidelines for HIV Testing 2008.*
www.bhiva.org/HIV-testing-guidelines.aspx

British Association for Sexual Health and HIV and MEDFASH (updated 2014) *Standards for the management of sexually transmitted infections (STIs).*
www.bashh.org/BASHH/About_BASHH/BASHH_Publications/BASHH/About_BASHH/BASHH_Publications.aspx?hkey=fd371e19-add9-435e-99dc-e54f0bda57ad
or
www.medfash.org.uk/publications

British Association for Sexual Health and HIV, British HIV Association, Faculty of Sexual and Reproductive Healthcare (2008) *UK guidelines for the management of sexual and reproductive health of people living with HIV infection.*
www.bhiva.org/SRH-guidelines.aspx

British HIV Association (2015) *BHIVA guidelines for the treatment of HIV-1-positive adults with antiretroviral therapy 2015*
www.bhiva.org/HIV-1-treatment-guidelines.aspx

British HIV Association (2015) *BHIVA guidelines on the use of vaccines in HIV-positive adults 2015*
www.bhiva.org/vaccination-guidelines.aspx

British HIV Association (2014) BHIVA guidelines for the management of HIV infection in pregnant women 2012 (interim review May 2014). *HIV Medicine* **15** (Suppl 4): 1-77
www.bhiva.org/pregnancy-guidelines.aspx

British HIV Association (2014) BHIVA guidelines for the management of hepatitis viruses in adults infected with HIV 2013 (updated September 2014)
www.bhiva.org/hepatitis-guidelines.aspx

British I IIV Association (2013) *Standards of care for people living with HIV 2013*
www.bhiva.org/standards-of-care-2013.aspx

British HIV Association (BHIVA) and Expert Advisory Group on AIDS (EAGA) (2014) *Position statement on the use of antiretroviral therapy to roduce HIV transmission. September 2014.*
www.bhiva.org/documents/Publications/Position-statement-on-the-use-of-antiretroviral-therapy-to-reduce-HIV%20transmission-sept2014.pdf

British Medical Association (2007) *Advance decisions and proxy decision-making in medical treatment and research – guidance from the BMA's Medical Ethics Department.*
www.bma.org.uk/advice/employment/ethics/mental-capacity/advance decisions-and-proxy-decision-making-in-medical-treatment-and-research

BNF Publications *British National Formulary* (HIV section)
www.medicinescomplete.com/mc/bnf/current/PHP78275-hiv-infection.htm

British Psychological Society, British HIV Association and MEDFASH (2011) *Standards for psychological support for adults living with HIV.*
www.bhiva.org/StandardsForPsychologicalSupport.aspx

Clutterbuck D, Flowers P, Barber T et al on behalf of the Clinical Effectiveness Group of the British Association for Sexual Health and HIV (BASHH) and the British HIV Association (BHIVA) (2012) UK national guideline on safer sex advice *International Journal of STD & AIDS* **23**(6): 381–388.
http://std.sagepub.com/content/23/6/381.abstract

Deutsche AIDS-Hilfe, European AIDS Treatment Group and International AIDS Society *Global database on HIV-specific travel and residence restrictions* (website)
www.hivtravel.org

eLearning for Healthcare *e-GP*
www.e-lfh.org.uk/programmes/general-practitioners

Faculty of Sexual and Reproductive Healthcare (2016) *UK Medical Eligibility Criteria for Contraceptive Use.*
www.fsrh.org/standards-and-guidance/uk-medical-eligibility-criteria-for-contraceptive-use

Faculty of Sexual and Reproductive Healthcare (2011, updated 2012) *Clinical Guidance: Drug Interactions with Hormonal Contraception.*
www.fsrh.org/documents/ceu-guidance-drug-interactions-with-hormonal-contraception-jan

General Medical Council *Confidentiality guidance: Disclosure after a patient's death.*
www.gmc-uk.org/guidance/ethical_guidance/confidentiality_70_72_disclosure_after_patient_death.asp

HIV in Europe (2012) *HIV Indicator Conditions: Guidance for Implementing HIV Testing in Adults in Health Care Settings.*
http://newsite.hiveurope.eu/Finalised-Projects/Guidance-HIV-Indicator-Conditions

Leake-Date H & Fisher M (2007) HIV Infection. In: Whittlesea C & Walker R (eds) *Clinical Pharmacy and Therapeutics* 4th Edition. Oxford: Churchill Livingstone.

Liverpool Drug Interactions Group *HIV drug interactions* (website).
www.hiv-druginteractions.org

MEDFASH *HIV TIPs (HIV Testing in Practice)*
www.medfash.org.uk/hiv-tips

NAM (2012) *HIV, stigma and discrimination.*
www.aidsmap.com/stigma

National AIDS Trust (2014) *Confidentiality in the NHS: Your Information, Your Rights. A guide on how personal confidential information on HIV is stored, used and shared within the NHS in England* www.nat.org.uk/HIV-in-the-UK/Key-Issues/Health-and-social-care/ Confidentiality-in-healthcare.aspx

National Institute for Health and Care Excellence (2013) *Guideline CG156: Fertility problems: assessment and treatment* www.nice.org.uk/guidance/CG156

National Institute for Health and Care Excellence (2011) *HIV testing: increasing uptake in black Africans* [PH33] www.nice.org.uk/Guidance/PH33

National Institute for Health and Care Excellence (2011) *HIV testing: increasing uptake in men who have sex with men* [PH 34] www.nice.org.uk/guidance/ph34

Public Health England *Country and PHE region HIV data tables* www.gov.uk/government/statistics/hiv-data-tables

Public Health England *HIV in the United Kingdom* reports www.gov.uk/government/statistics/hiv-in-the-united-kingdom

Public Health England *Immunisation against infectious disease* ('The Green Book'). www.gov.uk/government/collections/immunisation-against-infectious-disease-the-green-book

Public Health England (2014) *The Management of HIV infected Healthcare Workers who perform exposure prone procedures: updated guidance, January 2014* www.gov.uk/government/publications/hiv-infected-healthcare-workers-and-exposure-prone-procedures

Public Health England (2016) *NHS Infectious Diseases in Pregnancy Screening Programme Standards* www.gov.uk/government/publications/infectious-diseases-in-pregnancy-screening-programme-standards

UNAIDS (2014) *The Gap Report* www.unaids.org/en/resources/documents/2014/20140716_UNAIDS_gap_report

UNAIDS (2016) *Global AIDS Update 2016*
www.unaids.org/en/resources/documents/2016/Global-AIDS-update-2016

Adults and children estimated to be living with HIV, 2015. By WHO region.
Geneva: World Health Organization; 2016
http://gamapserver.who.int/mapLibrary/Files/Maps/HIV_all_2015.png

Section 6

Subject index

Subject index